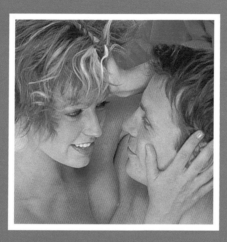

tantric
sex

dedication

I'd like to dedicate this book to my mother. I know it's not the sort of book you'd expect to be dedicated to someone's mother, but *none* of my books are the sort of books you'd normally dedicate to your mother.
So anyway – Hi, Ma ! This one's for you !

THIS IS A CARLTON BOOK

Text copyright © 2002 Suzie Hayman
Design and special photography copyright © 2002 Carlton Books Limited

This edition published by
Carlton Books Limited 2002
20 Mortimer Street
London W1T 3JW

A CIP catalogue record for this book is available from the British Library
ISBN 1 84222 472 7

Printed and bound in Italy

The author and publisher have made every effort to ensure that all information is correct and up to date at the time of publication. Neither the authors nor the publisher can accept responsibility for any accident, injury or damage that results from using the ideas, information or advice offered in this book.

The application and quality of essential oils is beyond the control of the above parties, who cannot be held responsible for any problems resulting from their use. Always follow the manufacturer's instructions and if in doubt, seek further advice.

Do not use essential oils without prior consultation with a qualified aromatherapist or medical doctor if you are pregnant, taking any form of medication, or if you suffer from oversensitive skin.

Editorial Manager: Judith More
Executive Editor: Zia Mattocks
Editor: Lisa Dyer
Design: DW Design
Picture Researcher: Marissa Keating
Production Manager: Garry Lewis

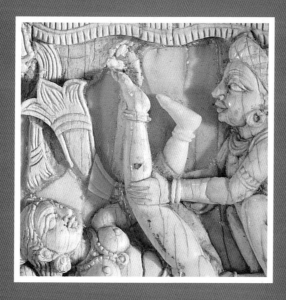

tantric
sex

learn the ancient art of
eastern lovemaking

Suzie Hayman

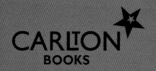

CARLTON
BOOKS

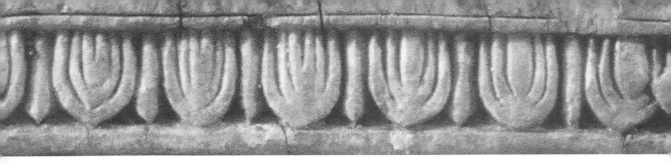

contents

INTRODUCTION
6

1 THE HISTORY OF
TANTRIC SEX
12

2 THE BASIC
PRINCIPLES
26

3 GETTING
IN TOUCH
52

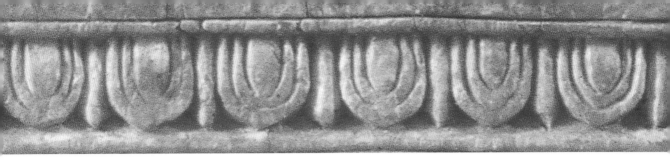

4

THE TANTRIC
RITUAL
78

5

TANTRIC SEX
POSITIONS
98

INDEX
126

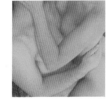

6

SEXUAL
ECSTASY
112

DIRECTORY &
ACKNOWLEDGMENTS
128

INTRODUCTION

Old World beliefs and New Age philosophies have become increasingly attractive in the last decade. Tantrism is one belief system that has attracted a lot of interest and it's easy to see why. Anything that seems to promise hour-long sex sessions and mind-blowing orgasms has to have something to recommend it, especially when blissed-out devotees who sing the praises of the Tantra and claim it has revitalized their relationships include such rock and movie stars

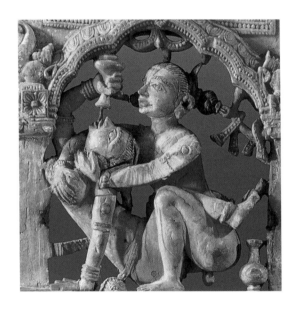

above: An erotic panel from an Indian temple shows sex as a glorious celebration of life and love.

as Sting and Woody Harrelson. You may have seen pictures of paintings or sculptures, or even the original works, showing couples or groups engaged in Tantric sex. One key element that may have drawn your interest is the evident pleasure and joy shown by those taking part. However, you might have been put off by what appears to be the commitment necessary to apply the Tantra to your life, both in mindfulness and time. The jargon may seem confusing and tongue-twisting; for example, do you have to know your 'chakra' from your 'yoni', your 'lingam' from your 'Kundalini'? The exercises may appear difficult and confusing; must you become adept at meditation, visualization, soul-gazing and obscure sexual positions to enjoy Tantric sex? What, you might ask, does a centuries-old religious practice have to do with modern-day life and loving? And even if you did want to take a leaf out of the Tantra's book, do you need the sort of free time and surroundings only available to millionaires? Or indeed, the sort of body only a film or rock star, or someone who can afford a personal trainer, may have? It clearly takes some effort to learn the techniques to get the best out of Tantric sex, and it sounds as if you may need to set quite a long period of time aside to learn. Tantra seems to call for plenty of space and privacy – can you make room for it in an ordinary, busy and crowded life? The average act of sex in the West is said to take ten minutes, while Tantric sex may let you in for at least an hour, if not several hours, of close involvement. Have you got the opportunities to do this in your full schedule?

Well, forget your preconceptions and reservations. Tantra may be based on beliefs and practices that are thousands of years old but, in fact, it has lessons that are totally up to date and have relevance today. Most important of all, anyone can incorporate lessons from the Tantra into their love life and gain enormously. Although the more you put in, the more you'll get out, it needn't take hours of study. With just a little planning and effort, you can turn your relationship and your sex life around from being OK, so-so or humdrum to dynamic, fulfilled and ecstatic.

One of the most important messages from the Tantra, which you can see depicted in Tibetan, Chinese and Indian art, is that sex is a natural, normal and beneficial part of life. Sadly, many of us in the West have grown up in a belief system that says sex is a distraction from the important things in life. We feel that in all but specific and quite rigid situations sex is sinful, dangerous and downright bad for you. The result is that a lot of us approach sex with a slightly guilty and hesitant air. We are scared of being hurt, we are frightened of being thought immoral and we are wary of showing any ignorance or incompetence. Sex is very much cordoned off as a special subject and a special event. The activity usually takes place in bed, after hours and with the lights out. Worst of all, we tend to adopt a rather 'hurry up and get it over with' approach to making love. Some people learn about sex behind the proverbial bicycle shed and many of us have our first experiences fearful that someone might walk in on us. This often means that we can get into the habit of doing it as quickly as possible. Western sex also tends to focus on results and results tend to mean orgasm. Everyone is chasing the Big O as the ultimate goal, wanting to get there as soon as they can.

below: This Indian miniature, depicting a chakra asana, exemplifies how traditional Eastern beliefs put sex firmly in the centre of life.

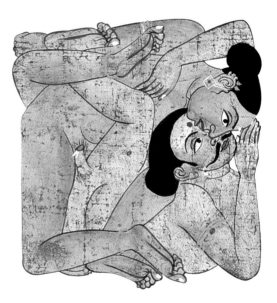

SEX IS A CELEBRATION

In contrast to our preconceived Western ideas concerning sex, Tantra has a very different message to give us: sex is a celebration, an integral part of life. A happy sex life is believed to be vital for your own personal wellbeing and for the development and fulfilment of a relationship. But more important, and perhaps more significant to us in the West, sex is seen as spiritual. Being sexual is a way of celebrating what we are and what we have been given. In fact, it is seen as a way of getting in touch with the spiritual forces – the gods and goddesses outside and within us. Tantrikas, practitioners of the Tantra, are positively encouraged to have sex as a way of showing devotion – both to each other and to the sacred universal force. Sex as a form of worship may seem quite strange and even shocking to Western minds, but it offers far more contentment than seeing sex as something to be ashamed about.

Even the words Tantrikas use can add something special to your love life. In the West, we tend to refer to sex acts and genitals either with medical-sounding terms, such as penis and vagina, or slang terms that we also use as insults and oaths. In the Tantric tradition, the words that describe our bodies, desires and sexual practices are beautiful and courteous. Using them encourages a respectful attitude towards your body, your sexual needs and desires, and your sexual relationship. It encourages you to honour and worship your partner – their body, their needs and their desires. There is nothing dirty or shameful in Tantric sex. A vagina is called a 'yoni', which means 'sacred space'. The penis is called a 'lingam', meaning 'wand of light'. A 'chakra' is an energy centre and 'Kundalini' is the life force and sexual energy. Tantrikas also use a word to mean both sex and love, which is 'kama'; the famous book the *Kama Sutra*, for instance, translates as 'Verses about Sex' or 'Verses about Love'. The same word is used whether you are talking about spiritual, emotional or physical matters. Significantly, what this means is that sex is love and love is sex, and both have an equal value and are to be prized.

below: Tantric tradition encourages respect and honour between partners, both in and out of the bedroom.

THE PLEASURE OF THE MOMENT

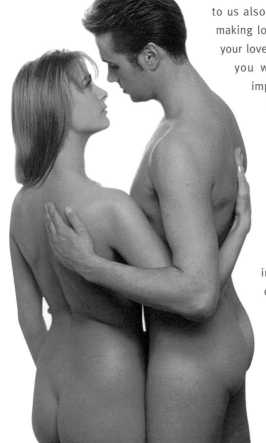

Seeing sex as a celebration of the gods and goddesses and their gifts to us also has some very specific advantages in the practice of making love. This is where Tantra can really enrich and open out your love and sex life. If you regard it as an act of worship, then you will understand that every aspect of the sex act is important. Your first touch, your kisses, your caresses and all the ways you explore and enjoy each other become just as important as what we may consider the end point, which is the orgasm. Indeed, in Tantra, orgasm is hardly considered the end of the act of love but just one more peak in a whole mountain range – and you are expected to enjoy the view as much as to conquer the summit! Tantric sex is not goal-oriented; instead, lovers are encouraged to take their time. Pleasing yourself and pleasing your partner are the most important things, and you can achieve this in so many delicious and various ways. Men are helped to last as long as possible, putting off the moment when they come, but enjoying repeated orgasmic sensations along the way. Women are encouraged to be multi-orgasmic,

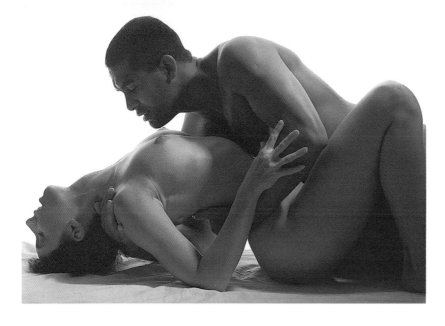

left: Passion and abandon are a healthy part of love, and couples are advised to take delight in the moment.

coming as many times as they wish. And men are encouraged to view a woman's orgasm as being of special benefit to them, too. Tantric sex is sex which acknowledges the pleasure of being 'in the moment', not sex which hurries onto one, single, explosive point. It tends to be a slow building up of pleasure that continues and may extend for quite some time, each succeeding moment being as pleasant as the one preceding it and the one after. Tantric sex also encourages experimentation and variety – no guilt or uncertainty is felt about using a wide range of positions or sex acts, provided they are carried out by loving and consenting adults. Couples are encouraged to let go in sex, to be abandoned and enthusiastic, and to enjoy the sensations sexual loving brings.

TANTRIC SEX AND TANTRIC LOVING

We live in an era when individuals are experiencing longer and healthier lives. A couple who commit themselves to each other at what has now become the average age of late twenties can look forward to at least 60 years together if they keep their 'till death do us part' promises. That's a lot of time to be living and loving in a single partnership, and it is why Tantra is of particular relevance to couples today. To make loving relationships work for that long, it helps to find ways of developing, deepening and indeed exploiting the intimacy and closeness that comes from long association.

One of the big advantages of the Tantra is that it does demand a certain amount of commitment and time. Couples who want to try Tantric sex will find that making it work in a hurried ten minutes, once every two weeks, is difficult. For it to be worthwhile, you have to operate together over a period of time. In striving to improve your sex life, however, you will find a spin-off benefit, which is that it enhances your relationship, too. But that does not mean to say that you will need to devote several hours a day in order to gain enormous advantages from it. Neither do you have to be engaged in sex rituals day after day to find that your emotional and sexual relationship improves. The exercises that you can carry out together will fit into any busy life, including family life, and will soon show results, helping you both in and out of bed. You don't have

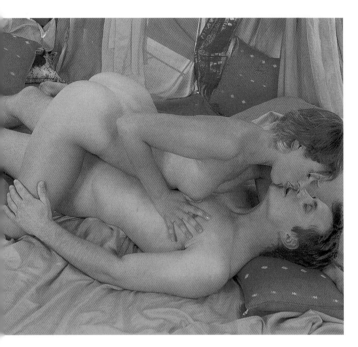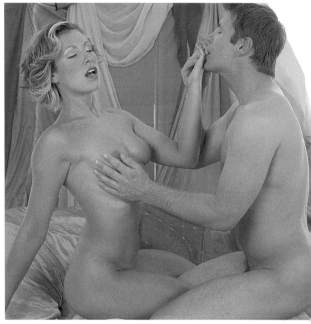

above left: Long, slow lovemaking allows you to explore and experiment, revealing your inner selves.

above right: You don't have to have penetration for sex to be explosive. Playfulness and sensual touching are erotic and stimulating.

to have penetrative sex to be involved in Tantric sex or Tantric loving. Simply being together and sharing interests and favourite pursuits, or enjoying kisses, loving caresses or nonsexual touches are as much a part of following the Tantra as the ground-moving sex for which it has become known.

The word 'Tantra' means to weave together, and it also means to extend. You can use Tantra to knit together your partnership, to bind yourselves closer together in an intimate and very sexy relationship. It can also extend your lives together and make your partnership last, as well as varied, exciting and vital. You won't need to think about having affairs to spice up and introduce something new into your life when you and your partner use the Tantra to bring you closer to each other and to enhance your sex life. Tantra teaches you to respect each other, to respect yourself and to respect sex, too. Sex is seen as being inextricably bound up in the way we view ourselves, our partners and our relationships, rather than being a separate and somewhat shameful activity. While it brings the sexual force into the whole of life, enriching much more than just the act itself, Tantra also encourages you to set aside special time to celebrate the rites of love. Tantric sex will show you how to enhance your loving time by making it more exciting and energizing. Most of all, as you might have heard, following the Tantra makes your sex life positively explosive!

TANTRA FOR ALL

You don't have to 'buy in' totally to the traditional Tantric belief system to make Tantric sex work for you. One person may see following the Tantra as two people getting in touch with the cosmos, embodying in themselves the spirit of Shiva and Shakti (see page 18), connecting with the dynamic energy in the universe and passing such force between them. Another may simply regard Tantric sex as a way of focusing on their partner and themselves, of paying each other undivided attention and communicating honestly and fully as they get closer and more intimate. Whichever way you view it, the result can be the same: a better relationship and an improved sex life.

below: Deep erotic kissing can be orgasmic, not just a prelude to penetration.

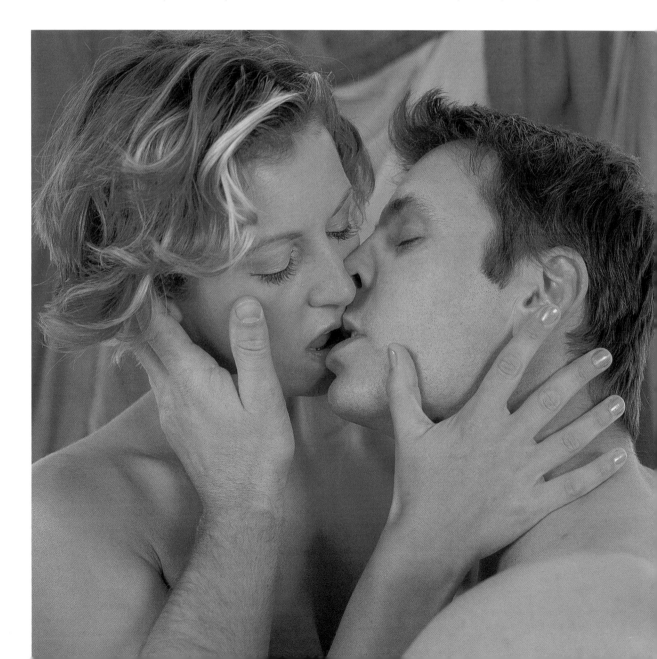

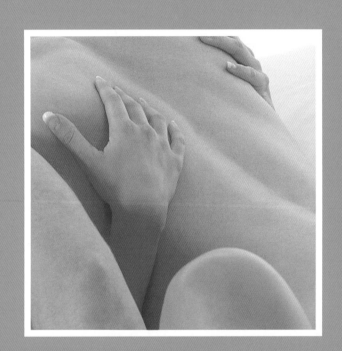

THE HISTORY OF TANTRIC SEX

1

BUDDHISTS AND HINDUS, FOR WHOM TANTRISM IS A SPIRITUAL AND PHILOSOPHICAL BELIEF SYSTEM, HAVE PRACTISED TANTRIC SEX FOR OVER 5,000 YEARS. PRACTITIONERS, KNOWN AS 'TANTRIKAS', CLAIM THAT TANTRIC SEX NOT ONLY SIGNIFICANTLY IMPROVES YOUR ALL-ROUND HEALTH BUT ALSO PROMOTES A SENSE OF INNER PEACE AND HARMONY.

Once they have tried Tantric sex, the after-effects for many people are startling and life-changing. Simply by doing what they do, and by carrying out the rituals that go before and after sex, you can heighten the anticipation and increase intimacy between yourself and your partner. These activities include pampering and cherishing each other, moving and dancing together and spending time enjoying each other's company. You can engage in the various practices and positions Tantrikas employ while making love, such as oral sex, a variety of sexual positions and methods of slowing down and extending the sex act, to make sex last longer and feel more sensational. This will certainly allow you and your partner to engage in the art of sexual ecstasy and let Tantra transform your love and sex lives. But you can go one better: by understanding the beliefs behind the actions, you can add an extra dimension to lovemaking. So what is Tantra and how and why does it work?

A WAY OF LIFE AND LOVE

above: This sculpture from the Khajuraho Temple in India shows an adorned couple on their quest to enlightenment.

Tantrism is a philosophy, a spiritual system and an art form, as well as a way of life. It is related to both Hinduism and Buddhism, and to the Chinese Tao, too. Although Tantrism is actually quite difficult to define and pin down, it has a lot in common with the Chinese Tao, in which one master said, 'the Tao you understand is not the real Tao'. What he meant by this was that the very act of analysing and explaining these particular beliefs actually changes and spoils them. Putting feelings and faith into words and reason is difficult; however, the real reason why Tantrism is confusing to Western eyes may be because it combines elements which we feel are contradictory – mainly, sex and spiritualism. In most of our belief systems, sex is seen as sinful, dangerous and, therefore, a bad thing. In the East, sex is often seen as an expression of the life force and doing it correctly is a way of connecting with the gods; it is, therefore, good. In the West, sex is regarded as something that distracts us from the quest for spiritual enlightenment, but in Eastern eyes, it *is* the quest for spiritual enlightenment!

Some religions chase after austerity, modesty and severity, seeing them as the price to pay for enlightenment. They turn their back on what feels pleasant, believing that to do you good, it must hurt, and that giving up pleasure in this world leads you to bliss in the next. Tantrikas believe sexual ecstasy is a taste of heaven and that if you heighten and extend the act of love, you deepen intimacy. But what is more important to them is that by doing this you become one with the universe and attain spiritual enlightenment. Tantrikas believe they will achieve higher spiritual awareness by experiencing all the senses in the here and now. The argument is that if the gods created the world and us, they made it to be enjoyed and celebrated, not ignored. However, Tantra isn't simply do-as-you-want, out-of-control pleasure-seeking. Participants have to control and channel sexual indulgence to make creative, positive use of it.

A Sanskrit word, 'Tantra' can be translated into what seems to be a bewildering number of different ways, some apparently contradictory. It means 'to expand and to spin out', but also 'to weave together'. In fact, the two go hand-in-hand because what Tantra does is to put those who practise it at the centre of the universe, connected to the gods and all things. Sex is placed at the centre of a healthy life, which includes a happy relationship. Indeed, sex is seen as the act that knits it all together. Tantric sex helps to prolong lovemaking in order to attain a perfect sense of bliss and union with yourself, your partner and the cosmos. While practising it, you *become* the god and goddess, Shiva and Shakti, and experience the energies and the power they personify.

In Tantra, the world is seen as something created by the gods. According to myths, at some time in the distant past, these gods were attacked by a demon and only prevailed by combining all their energies, which were channelled through Vishnu, the Hindu god of creation, and Shiva, the personification of thought and consciousness. These energies appeared as streams of flames which flowed out and then solidified into the shape of a goddess. Tantra sees our own personal universes as a battleground in which a similar war is fought day after day, with energy that can be transformed into healing or destructive forces. Each of us is composed of both male and female attributes. Tantric sex allows us to bring these out and to purify, celebrate and worship them, in ourselves and in our partners. Sex is not seen as being simply a selfish act of pleasure but a way of controlling the energy of the universe for virtuous use, and of finding your inner self and your place in the great cycle of being.

The Kama Sutra

Although Tantra is much older in the history of Sanskrit literature, the book that is taken as the standard text on sexual love was written around 1,800 years ago, sometime between 100 and 300 AD. This is the *Kama Sutra*, the 'Verses on Love/Sex', written by the Hindu philosopher Vatsyayana. He advocated that adherents should master their sexual impulses and that the best way to do this was to become a student and expert in the arts of love. He believed that you could win material, spiritual and amorous success in life if you conquered sexuality rather than let it rule you. According to Vatsyayana, anyone who preserves their virtue or religious merit (dharma), secures wealth (artha) and practises sensual gratification (kama) shall be free and in control of their own destiny. The more times you have Tantric sexual union, the stronger and healthier and the more in control of yourself and your fate you become.

KUNDALINI ENERGY

Tantrikas believe that the physical universe as we see it is matched by an invisible one of energy and power. Just as the outer material world contains a hidden, inner core, so they believed our bodies had potent, hidden spiritual and sexual energy forces within. Tantra is all about getting in touch with the invisible cosmos by mobilizing the hidden forces within ourselves. In Tantric belief, there is a vital sexual and spiritual force called Kundalini, or 'prana', which lies inside every person's body. This was visualized, and shown in paintings, as a serpent coiled around the base of the spine. It can be activated by meditation or through sexual activity, when it rises up the body, passing from one energy vortex to another to reach the uppermost one. When it reaches a point at the crown of the head, the Tantrika will experience a sense of bliss called 'samadhi'.

According to Tantric belief, the energy of the universe and of ourselves enters into and exits out of vortexes or gates that run in a line all the way along

below left: An illustration from Theosophica Practica depicts the seven chakras, or energy gates, of the body.

below right: Meditation can activate Kundalini energy and help you to achieve an enlightened state.

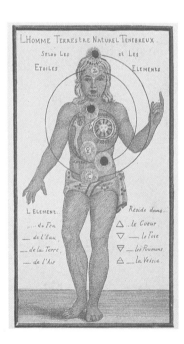
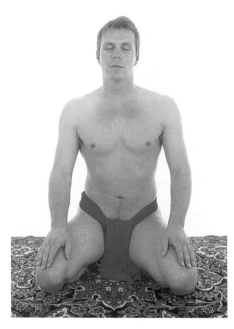

the body. These are called 'chakras'. Hindus, Buddhists and Taoists all agree on the existence and function of these energy centres; however, they tend to disagree on the number of chakras. Some traditions say there are seven chakras, while others list only five, and others still many more. Even Western philosophers, such as the psychologist, Carl Jung, believe in their existence. Just as organs, such as the liver, kidneys and heart, have specific jobs to do in the smooth working of the physical body, so the chakras are believed to have particular roles to perform in receiving and refining the life force, or energy. The chakras run from the base of the spine up to the crown of the head. Modern practitioners point out that the chakras' position also corresponds with various important hormone-producing glands in the physical body, and that's why many Eastern methods of healing, such as massage, are worked along the chakras.

In Tantric belief, there is also an equivalent life force corresponding to the circulatory system. Just as veins and arteries carry blood around the body, so the 'nadis' transports the stream of energy around the body from one chakra to another. Tantrikas use yoga and sex to open up the chakras and channel energy along the nadis to achieve 'samadhi', or bliss. There is one other special point, called 'bindu', which is located on the back of the skull where the hair naturally spirals outward. This is the reason why monks shave their heads: to leave a bald spot at the critical point and let their energy come to the surface.

The Seven Chakras

The First Gate: Muladhara
Near the adrenal glands – the perineum in men and inside the vagina in women – this gate, or chakra, is envisaged as a red flower with four petals.

The Second Gate: Svadhisthana
Found near the sexual glands – the ovaries in the woman and the prostate in the man – this chakra is envisaged as an orange flower with six petals.

The Third Gate: Manipura
Lying near the solar plexus, close to the pancreas, this gate is envisaged as a yellow flower with ten petals.

The Fourth Gate: Anahata
Near the heart and thymus, this is envisaged as a green 12-petalled flower.

The Fifth Gate: Vishuddi
Positioned in the throat near the thyroid gland, this chakra is envisaged as a sky blue flower with 16 petals.

The Sixth Gate: Ajna
Located at the point between the eyebrows near the pineal gland, this chakra is envisaged as an indigo blue flower with two petals.

The Seventh Gate: Sahasrara
Located at the top of the head, this highest chakra is envisaged as a purple or white flower with 1,000 petals.

MALE AND FEMALE ENERGY

In Tantric practice, sexual partners use various means to reflect the cosmos in themselves. Men become the god Shiva, who is the personification of the male force. Women become the goddess Shakti, who personifies the female force. Through intimate contact, both can share male and female sexual energies. In Tantric belief, both genders possessed various amounts of what was seen as male and female energy. Female energy, however, is the power that is stronger and most desirable and women possess more of it. While male energy is regarded as active, powerful and strong, it is also considered to be passive and only brought into reality if worked through the female principle. In fact, the whole aim of sexual connection in Tantrism is for the man to absorb his partner's female energy and so release his own. The longer a couple make love, the more orgasms the woman achieves and the more often the man can delay his, the more energy he will absorb.

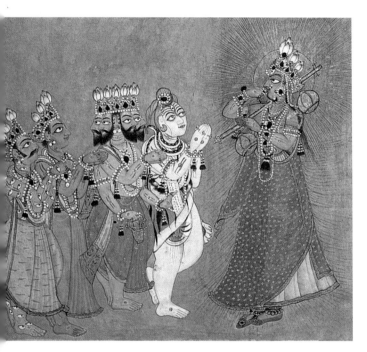

above: Women are cherished as personifying the more powerful female force in this Indian miniature of the gods worshipping Devi.

While the societies that revered the Tantra were also quite sexist and male-ruled, belief in the power of the female meant that women were seen as important and to be cherished, if only so that men could get what they wanted from them – sexual union. You can only share energies if both parties are wholly involved, willing and happy about the exchange. These energies can't be wrested or taken by force. Because the woman's sexual energy was so coveted, this resulted in a higher status for women in cultures following the Tantric principles than might otherwise have been the case.

In Tantric texts, such as the *Kama Sutra*, men are encouraged to honour, cherish and love their partners. Even when, in the section on seduction, the author of the *Kama Sutra* gives advice on how the man has his way with the wife of an enemy to get back at him, it is still seduction, not rape, that is being discussed. Although, historically, Tantrism focused on male needs and desires, it resulted in women being worshipped and valued. Today, with the importance of equality between the sexes being acknowledged, Tantrism is seen as a meeting of equals to share the life force and pleasure, and a way to learn from each other. At its root remains the overriding necessity that drove the Tantra, which is that for the man to achieve his ends – his orgasm and increased energies, he had to first give his partner a very good time indeed!

Exchanges of energy

Because Tantrikas believed that sexual bliss moved energy through, and in and out, of the chakras, the idea was to align chakras and therefore exchange energies between the couple, either by having sexual intercourse, embracing closely or simply sitting close to each other. By concentrating and focusing while becoming aroused, sexual energy could be passed through the chakras, from one area of the body to another, and from one body to another. The reason why Tantric sex involves so many different sexual positions is because aligning various chakras helps to move sexual energy around and passes different energies from one person to another.

Furthermore, there is a traditional Hindu belief that the body fluids produced through intercourse have certain powers in themselves. Tantrikas were among the first to recognize the existence of female ejaculation and the G-spot. Without argument, men ejaculate; that is to say, they produce semen when they orgasm. However, excellent evidence exists to prove that many women do so, too, even though some people still have their doubts. Not all women ejaculate, and those who do don't necessarily do so every time they climax. However, a growing number of women report that they produce generous amounts of fluid from their vagina as they orgasm, and research has shown that this is neither urine nor simply vaginal fluid. Eastern sources took female ejaculate for granted, even giving it a name. Male semen is called 'bindu' and female ejaculate is called 'amrita'. Since men tend to become tired and lose their erections after orgasm, the belief evolved that a man shedding his semen was akin to him losing his 'essence' and strength. Because women tend to be able, and more than willing, to continue to have sex after climaxing, and can go on to multiple orgasms, it seemed obvious that women were the ones with more sexual energy and that this was concentrated in their sexual fluids.

Tantric sex, then, seeks to let men preserve and concentrate their sexual energies by delaying or holding off ejaculation. At the same time, it strives to encourage the woman to achieve as many orgasms as possible. Traditional thought is that the woman loses nothing by spending her amrita, but her partner only gains by reabsorbing his own energy and absorbing her energy too, which is far more expansive and powerful than his own and comes to him through her amrita. In addition to this, if Tantric sex is not done properly, the male loses by giving away all his strength and energy to the female. In this context, doing it improperly means sex is quick and hurried, and the man is allowed to come before the woman has done so at least once, if not several times. If the man can hold off his own orgasm until after the woman comes, both gain; if, instead, he lets go too quickly and she misses out, both lose. Needless to say, most women are only too happy to allow their partners to 'steal' their sexual energy in this way!

The way of the Tao

About 500–600 years after Vatsyayana wrote the *Kama Sutra*, Tantrism spread from India to China, and the Chinese concentrated on and perfected techniques to prevent male ejaculation. In Taoism, the idea that a man can harvest sexual energy from the woman by putting off or even avoiding ejaculation altogether is very important. Taoists believed that women had much larger sexual appetites and the capacity for multiple orgasms and hence had more sexual energy – yin energy to his yang. It was assumed that a woman would experience a number of orgasms without any physical, emotional, or sexual harm and still be connected to the goddess inside herself, while men would collapse and fall asleep, so losing their connection to the universe. For that reason, men are encouraged to bring a woman to as many orgasms as possible while delaying or even refraining from their own orgasm so that the man can benefit from the woman's energy. The longer a man could remain within his partner, and the more orgasms he could encourage her to have, the more yin energy he would absorb. Taoists discovered that if pressure was applied to the spot between the scrotum and anus, called the perineum, just as the man felt he was about to ejaculate, he would be able to orgasm but delay ejaculation.

The vital forces held in reserved male semen concentrate around the first and second chakras, Muladhara and Svadhisthana. Tantric practitioners believed that the semen travelled directly to the brain and that a rush of sexual energy flowed through the chakras up to the crown chakra, the Sahasrara. American sex therapists, Masters and Johnson, rediscovered these sexual practices in the late 1970s, so sparking off renewed interest in the rituals and practices of Tantrism. They recorded that it was indeed possible for a man to train himself to experience all the pleasure of orgasm without ejaculation, thus enabling him to enjoy multiple orgasms and to last longer so his partner could do so, too.

THE SIXTY-FOUR ARTS

top left and right: Activating all five senses adds to sexual satisfaction. Feeding your partner by hand and simply sharing food and wine can arouse erotic feelings.

centre: Challenging the mind will bring a couple closer together and allow both of you to discover different facets of your personalities.

below left and right: Dancing and moving together, one of the Sixty-four Arts, sets the blood and juices flowing.

To have Tantric sexual intercourse, you do need to follow fairly strict guidelines. The sexual act itself takes place as part, and only part, of a whole experience called the Tantric Sex Ritual. A couple build up to actually having sex by first awakening all the senses – touch, taste, scent, sound and sight. They delight in the beauty of their surroundings and the pleasure they take in each other. Both are then tantalized through preparing and sharing food and drink together, breathing in pleasant perfumes, listening to music and hearing each other talk. They may challenge each other's mind by playing games, and get the blood as well as the juices flowing by moving together in dance. In Vatsyayana's day, every respectable man and woman was expected to be well versed in the Sixty-four Arts. Just as women in the novelist Jane Austen's day, the early 1800s, were

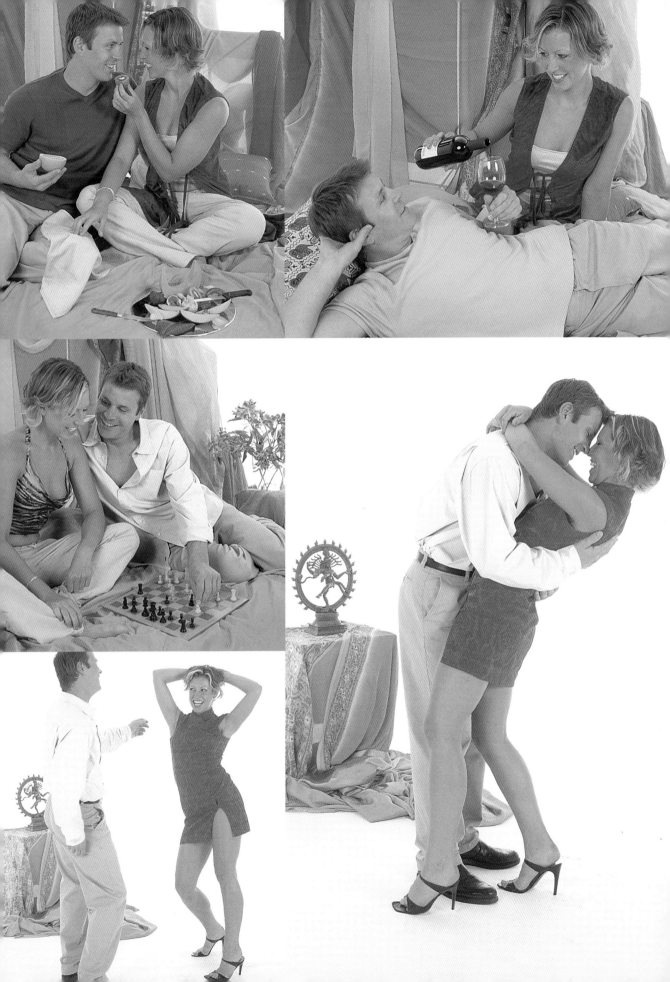

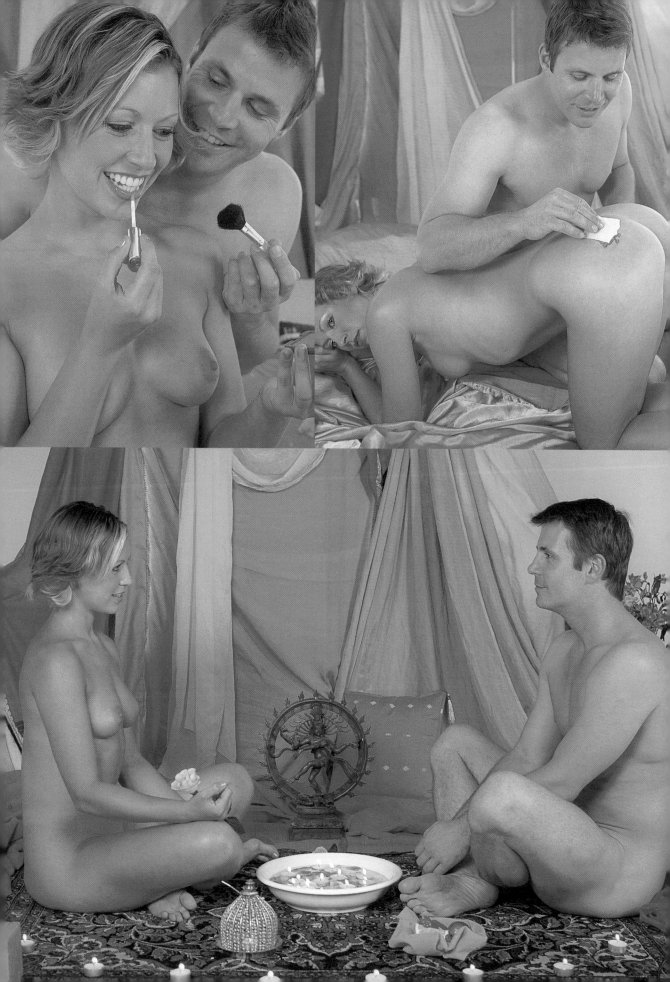

expected to be able to play the piano, sing, dance and paint, so both men and women in Vatsyayana's time were expected to be able to do a host of things to charm each other and pass the time. They would be skilled in writing and drawing, painting and making stained glass, sewing, reading, composing and reciting poetry, sculpture, gymnastics, flower arranging, making perfumes and jewellery, gardening, solving problems, languages, etiquette, carpentry, magic, chemistry, mineralogy, gambling, architecture, logic, making charms, religious rites, household management, mimicry and disguise, physical sports and martial arts. When preparing to make love, they would amuse and entertain each other with some of the Sixty-four Arts. These would include arranging the room so it looked attractive, dancing for or with their partner, playing games, adorning each other with tattoos, putting on make-up, preparing food and drink, serving each other and making each other feel welcome. Sex was only one aspect of the experience, and not the most important or the last one.

left: The Sixty-four Arts teach you to adorn yourself and your partner and to focus upon them completely.

MANTRAS

Since the goal is to increase concentration of female energy in the man, Tantrikas need to take a disciplined approach and to follow ritual when making love. Sex should only take place when both partners are sexually excited, and the man tries not to ejaculate at all or does so only after the woman has had at least one, or preferably multiple, orgasms. Couples are advised to employ self discipline and sexual positions and variations to prevent the man from ejaculating prematurely – and this doesn't mean after a few minutes, but a few hours. Partners are expected to align chakras, to visualize and activate the Kundalini force through chanting, movement and meditation, and to allow life-force energy to flow easily through these centres and systems.

below: Setting a candle-lit, intimate stage for your time together first will enhance the Tantric experience.

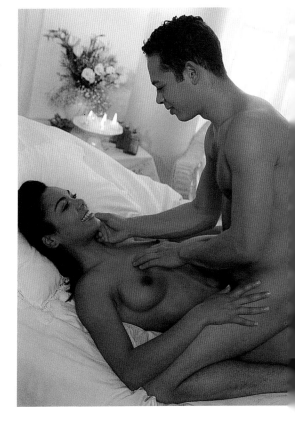

To open up the chakras and direct energy round the body, Tantrikas use mantras. These are sounds that resonate and bring both sexes to the correct pitch of emotion and sexual feeling. Perhaps the most well known mantra is *om mani padme aum*. Translated literally this means 'the jewel is in the lotus', and it is an image many people use in meditation. However, in Tantric sex it has a more specific meaning, which is 'the lingam is in the yoni' (the penis is in the vagina). At the same time, Tantrikas fix their minds on a visual representation of the chakra they want to open: a red flower with four petals if it is the first gate, Muladhara, that they want to energize, or an orange flower with six petals if it is the second gate, Svadhisthana. As the chakras

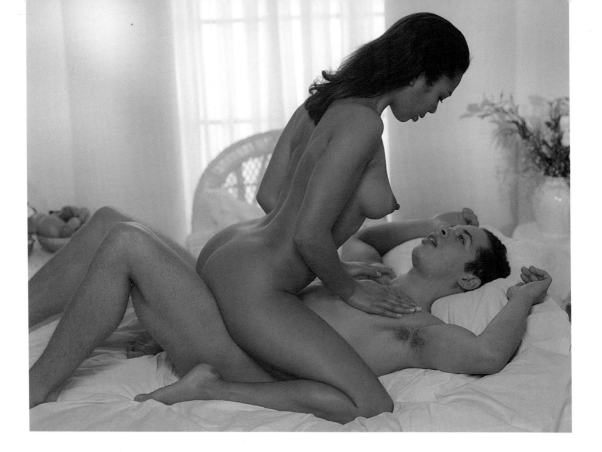

and nadis are energized, Tantrikas will notice such sensations as feelings of warmth, tingling of the skin, vibrations and pressure at various points. Partners need to be initiated into and to understand 'mudras' – the positions of their bodies and hands during lovemaking – in order to open or close the chakras and lead them both to total bliss.

THE COSMIC CYCLES

Following Tantric sex rituals has more far-reaching consequences than simply allowing you and your partner to have sensationally satisfactory sex. There is a universal dimension to it, too. Hindus and Buddhists believe that history goes in cycles. Each cycle is less pure than the one before and each one begins and ends in ruin. They believe we are approaching the end of the fourth and last era, the most violent and destructive of all. Tantric belief is that we should not avoid the powerful forces personified in sex but, instead, 'ride the tiger'. We should work with the forces that can become destructive and transform them into positive, healing energies. For that reason, practising Tantric sex is not only beneficial for individuals but for the universe at large, too. The belief is that each and every time you and your partner join with each other in Tantric sex, you won't just be giving yourselves extreme pleasure: you may also be contributing to world peace and the preservation of the cosmos! In order to follow the rituals involved in Tantric sex, you do need to know a fair amount about the basic underlying principles, and this is covered in the next chapter.

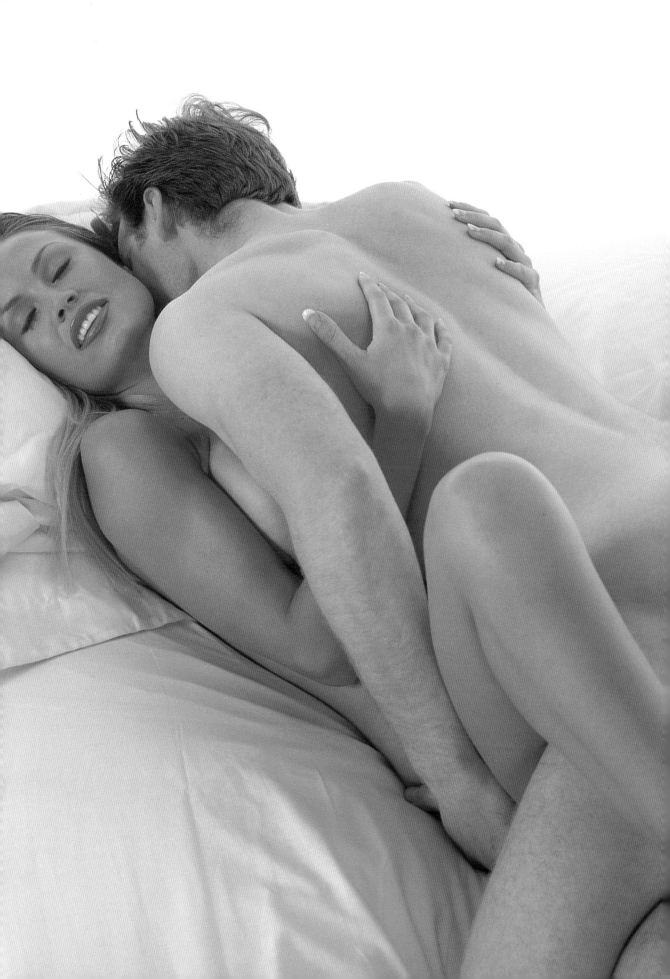

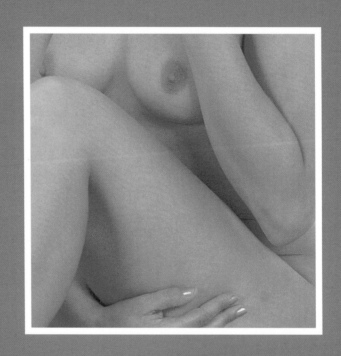

THE BASIC PRINCIPLES

2

TANTRIC SEX PROMISES ENORMOUS REWARDS FOR YOUR SEX LIFE AND YOUR RELATIONSHIP OVERALL. TO GET THE REWARDS. HOWEVER. YOU DO NEED TO PUT IN A BIT OF EFFORT FIRST. HERE ARE NINE BASIC PRINCIPLES TO RECOGNIZE AND EMPLOY. WHICH WILL HELP YOU ON YOUR WAY TO MORE FULFILLING AND ENRICHED LOVEMAKING.

Once you are aware of the importance of the basic principles of Tantric sex, and have some knowledge of, and practise in, them, your quest for enlightenment and exquisite sex will become much easier. To transform their lovemaking and enhance spiritual connection, Tantrikas use ritual, meditation, breathing, mantras, visualization, movement, yoga, touch and massage.

These are the basic philosophies and practices, and each one will add to your experience. Although you do not have to be expert in every one to make Tantric sex a part of your life and love, it certainly helps to have some practise in them all. In trying them out, you and your partner will find yourselves gaining or becoming adept in another vital skill – communicating and getting to know each other on a fuller, deeper level.

RITUALS

below: Meditation, one of the first basic rituals of Tantric sex, is a preparation for action.

Tantric rituals make sex a very special event, and in doing so, each Tantrika conveys the message to their partner that they value themselves, their lover and the time they spend together. By making a great deal of the lovemaking experience, you avoid fencing off sex, or saying that it is separate and apart from real life. Instead, you affirm that sex has the power to elevate and energize you, your partner and your relationship, not just while you are making love but before, after and throughout your day. Performing a ritual means doing things in a set way: formally and with the respect due to something important and special. By doing so, you approach sex aware that it is central to self image and needs, and you acknowledge that sex has the potential to heal and develop, to change and transform you. But this doesn't mean that you always need to make love with Tantric ritual. There may be times when you want to put aside the forms and the demands of Tantric sex for something that's altogether quicker, easier and different. But practising Tantric sex and making it part of yourself and your relationship can work a transformation that might surprise and delight you.

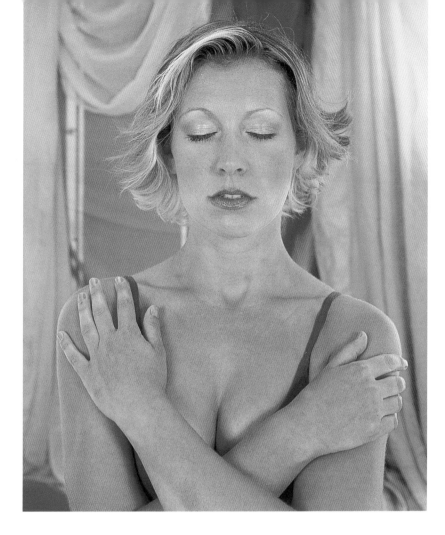

left: Concentrating on your breathing while meditating will help you to achieve whole body awareness.

Many of the things you do in the Tantric Sex Ritual may go on to become second nature and an essential part of your lovemaking. Rituals involve creating a special and thus sacred space for lovemaking, and concentrating on your body so that it is ready and prepared for Tantric sex. This may involve meditation, correct breathing, and the use of sound, movement and touch to focus you on the time ahead together. Such practices will prepare and speed you on your way to enjoying a very special experience (see also chapter 4, pages 78–97).

MEDITATION

Meditation is a misunderstood and much-maligned exercise. To learn what it is, how you do it, what it can do for you and why it works, you first need to understand what it is not. Meditation is not sleeping, relaxing or going into a trance. If you find yourself falling asleep when you try to meditate, the best thing to do is to leave your attempt until later! Tuck yourself up in bed and have a good sleep – you are obviously tired and in no state to do it.

Neither is meditation simply relaxing. Relaxation techniques are often used to assist people with stress and anxiety, but what they do is to help you control your breathing, loosen your muscles and generally slow down. While this can

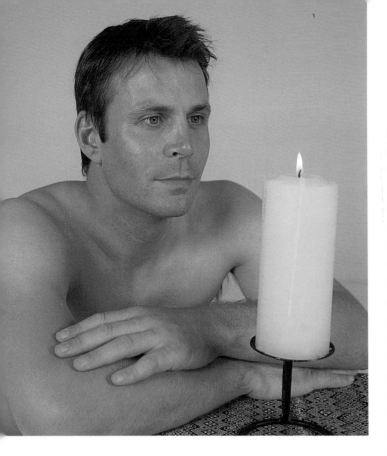

be very helpful and it's also good for you, it isn't meditating. Meditating can lead you to feeling relaxed and rested afterwards, but it's not just a case of chilling out and letting go. Nor does it put you into a trance whereby you drift away, unaware of yourself and your surroundings. Meditation itself is actually a very active state, one in which you look for and manipulate changes in your body and in your emotions, too. It is all about concentration. When you meditate, you focus all your attention and regard on one thing only. It can be an object, a sound or a sensation in your own body. In meditating, you sink yourself into the subject of your attention to get to know it fully. You examine it as it is, and watch for changes and alterations. It doesn't matter if nothing happens, or a great

above: *While meditating, learn to live in the moment and watch for change.*

deal occurs. What you are trying to do is to observe the moment in time as each second goes by. You can meditate by gazing at a candle or a pool or stream of water. Some people meditate by noticing texture: holding a fabric or stroking clothing, a smooth pebble or a flower and concentrating on the feel – whether it is soft, smooth, rough, scratchy, warm or cool. In readying yourself for Tantric sex, it often helps to start by observing your own breathing patterns.

BREATHING

Noticing your own breathing is a common meditation technique and perhaps the most useful one to begin with. You can do this alone or with your partner. First, make your surroundings as cosy as possible. Wear loose and comfortable clothing and ensure that the room is warm and you feel safe and protected. Set aside the time and make sure no-one will interrupt you – and that the phone is off – or your answering machine is switched on but you can't hear it!

Settle down in a comfortable position. You need to sit with your back straight, but you do not need to be in the lotus position (where you sit cross-legged with each foot on the opposite thigh). This takes some practise and you do need to be lithe and flexible. You can sit with crossed legs, or in a half-lotus position, which is where one foot is raised to rest on the opposite thigh and the other is placed beneath the opposite leg. Or simply sit in a chair. Use cushions, pillows and blankets to prop yourself up if you so desire, and make yourself as comfortable as possible. You do need to support yourself because you will be sitting still for at least 20 minutes. Make sure that you are sitting firmly on your backside, not perched on the edge of a chair or in any other precarious position, and that the rest of your body is not touching anything. Leaning back against a sofa or lying on a bed is not the ideal position for meditating because you need to be able to focus deeply on sensations and touches, and having a firm presence against your back may interfere with concentration. If the room is not as warm as you would like, or if sitting still makes you feel cold, drape a soft shawl or blanket across your shoulders.

Once you have closed your eyes and focused on your breathing, two things may soon compete for your attention. One is that it can be hard to focus on one thing at a time. You may find your mind drifts off after every little sound or smell, or that thoughts of day-to-day concerns needing your attention intrude. Did you turn off the iron? Do you need to buy milk? Have you forgotten to ring your mother? But none of this matters. The idea behind meditation is to live in the moment, to focus on something and then recognize and know it. Each moment succeeds the last and each one is complete in itself. That each moment of meditation is punctuated by thinking about other things doesn't really matter and will not detract from your concentration.

The other thing you may notice is how dynamic and busy even a body at rest seems to be. You may have thought nothing much happens when you close your eyes and drift off. But when you meditate, you soon realize that this is not so – and that's a large part of the point of meditation. If you close your eyes and listen, you'll soon hear plenty of sounds: your heart thumping, blood swishing through your arteries, and tendons and joints popping and creaking as you shift or move in place. You will hear the breath go in and out of your nose and mouth and lungs. You will also become aware of movement – of fingers, toes and limbs twitching, of eyes blinking, of the blood moving around, of lungs inflating and heart muscles throbbing.

You will begin to become aware of how elements change and progress. As you meditate, you may find your heart slows down and breathing becomes more regular. You may begin to notice how it feels to take a breath – the sensation of air coming into your nostrils, down your windpipe and into your lungs. So concentrate on this – the sensation of breathing in and breathing out. Consider the fact that you have to go on breathing to live. Breathing speeds up if you exert yourself by walking quickly, running or cycling, and it slows down when you are at rest. You may hold your breath when you are scared, angry or surprised; you may blow it out when you want to shout, scream or cry, but breath is life and you can't do without it. You can't stop it, but you can control it. Steadying your breathing when you are upset or suffering a panic attack can often bring a measure of calm and helps stop hyperventilation. In other words, control your breathing and you control your state of mind, too.

Deep breathing exercise

Being aware of your breathing is the first entry into meditation. Once you have followed your breath down your windpipe, into your lungs and out, move your focus on and become aware of other movement and sensation in your body. Concentrate on a fingertip or toe, or a spot between your shoulder blades. Can you feel it? How does it feel? Is it warm, cold, smarting or tickling? Direct your awareness to this place, on or in your body, and you may find the spot begins to tingle, or to feel cold or warm, as you focus on it. Or you may discover your attention is called to an area that is feeling sensation. Once you home in on it, you may find the sensations intensify or recede.

Just as you followed your breath down your body and out again, follow sensations around the veins and arteries, along the skin and through the bones. Trace, with your mind, the connections and lines of your physical body as you breathe in and out and slowly, patiently, follow your awareness. As you breathe, you may also become aware of your sense of smell – your ability to detect scents and perfumes, aromas and odours. Some people use fragrance to meditate upon, burning incense sticks or using a vaporizer to release the perfume from fragrant oils. Breathe in the scents and let them permeate into your body. Examine the feelings and memories each fragrance calls up.

MANTRAS

As well as concentrating on your body – your breathing, the ebb and flow of your blood and the beat of your heart – it often helps to concentrate on a sound. You could listen to water trickling, such as a stream or a water feature in your garden if you have one, or a CD or tape of running water. Many people find their meditation is helped enormously by having a mantra. A mantra is a word, phrase or collection of syllables that may mean something to you, or are just sounds. You say your mantra slowly, deliberately and repeatedly, like a chorus in a song. You can meditate on the meaning of the word or phrase, or you can use the sound simply to stop yourself from thinking about anything in particular.

The simplest, but often thought to be the most potent, Hindu mantra is 'om'. This is said with three distinct separate sounds: aah, ou and mm, the whole making up a word best written as 'aum'. Say it so it resonates and echoes, and listen carefully to the vibrations it sets up in yourself. One of the most common and popular Tantric mantras is *om mani padme aum*. Literally, this translates as 'the jewel is in the lotus', which is an arresting and beautiful image. You may remember that the Sanskrit word for vagina is 'yoni', meaning 'sacred space', and penis is 'lingam', which is 'wand of light'. The female genitals are also often likened to a lotus flower, and the glans of the penis to a jewel. So *om mani padme aum* can also be interpreted as another way of saying, 'the lingam is in the yoni' or the 'penis is in the vagina' – an image worth contemplating while preparing to have Tantric sex with your partner.

VISUALIZATION

In meditating you can concentrate your mind by focusing on a sight, such as a flickering candle flame, or use your imagination and your mind's eye to summon up an image. In Tantric tradition, one of the purposes of meditation is to allow you to prepare to move energy up from chakra to chakra, to achieve bliss, and to take in energy from the cosmos and exchange it with your partner. Meditation helps to open and purify the chakras and nadis – the energy gates and channels through which energy moves. This allows life-force energy to flow easily through your body, and to and from your partner. Unlike veins and arteries, chakras and nadis cannot be seen, but Tantrikas believe they can most certainly be felt as they become energized. As you focus on the energy circulating within your body, you may begin to feel warm and cold, and locate tingling, throbbing and pulsing sensations. When you start, these sensations may seem to come from all over your body and may be spread out and wide-ranging. The feelings that call your attention may seem to be different each time you meditate, and even to move as you sit and focus. As you practise more, however, you may find you can narrow them down to one area and keep your focus on one point. It often helps to visualize, to imagine in your mind's eye the point you want to concentrate upon, to become energized by your attention and efforts, and to 'see' the changes you want to take place.

Sit down in a comfortable position and make sure your back is straight. You can cross your legs, with your backside supported by a cushion or on the floor. Take the half- or full lotus

below: Use your imagination to see the chakras and nadis of your body, concentrating on the coloured flower images of the chakras.

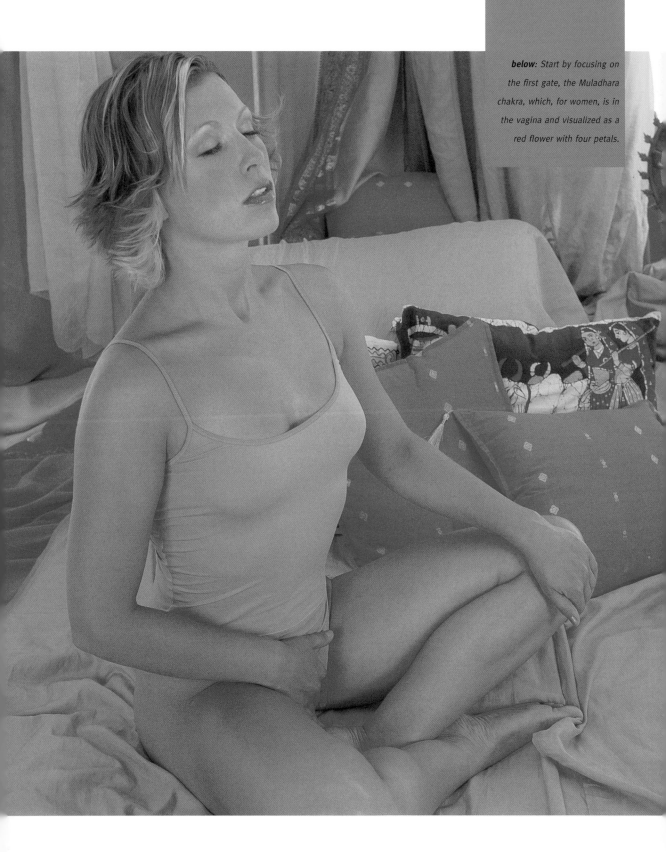

below: Start by focusing on the first gate, the Muladhara chakra, which, for women, is in the vagina and visualized as a red flower with four petals.

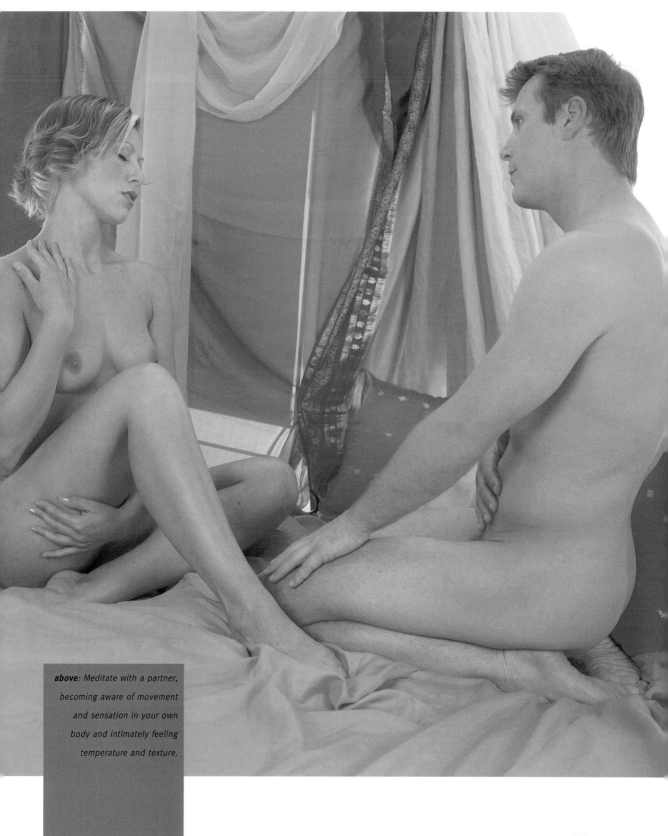

above: Meditate with a partner, becoming aware of movement and sensation in your own body and intimately feeling temperature and texture.

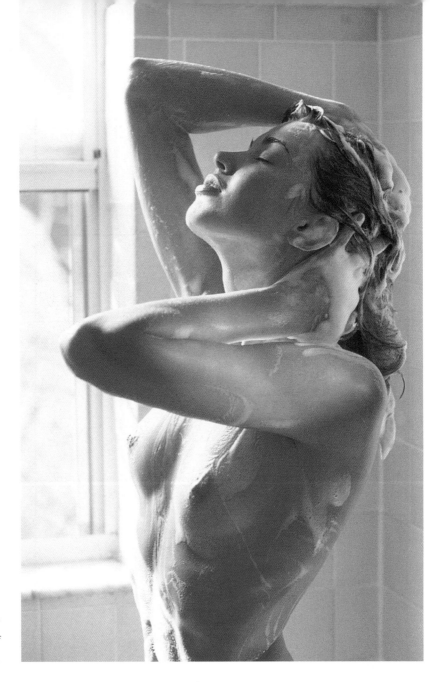

right: As you inhale, pull the breath of life inside yourself and experience the energy.

position (see pages 40–41). If you find this uncomfortable, sit upright in a chair, but move forward slightly so your backside is placed firmly on the seat, but you are not touching the back of the seat.

In Sanskrit, chakra means 'wheel', and you can imagine each chakra as a wheel of light, each with its own colour. But this wheel is also formed in the shape of a flower and each chakra has a certain number of petals. Start by focusing on Muladhara chakra, the lowest chakra. When moving energy and meditating, you should always start by moving energy up, from the lowest chakra to the highest, from Muladhara towards Sahasrara. Then, to complete the circle, bring your focus back down again from Sahasrara to Muladhara, and repeat the process as long as you desire.

Visualizing the Chakras

1 Concentrate on the perineum, the point midway between your scrotum or anus, if you are a man, or the inside of your vagina if you are a woman. Be aware of any sensations. The Muladhara chakra is the root chakra and is associated with the earth and basic survival needs. It is also the centre of sexuality for the man. Picture the Muladhara chakra as a red flower with four petals and concentrate on this image for three to four minutes. Imagine the energy gate glowing with a red light.

2 Now move up to the second chakra, Svadhisthana, which is found near the sexual glands: the ovaries in the woman, or the prostate in the man. It is associated with emotions, friendliness, intuition and creativity, and is the centre for female sexuality. Visualize this as an orange flower with six petals and imagine it glowing with an orange light.

3 After three to four minutes, move to the third gate, Manipura, located at the solar plexus. This is envisaged as a yellow flower with ten petals and is associated with intelligence and expressiveness, power and authority. Imagine it glowing with a yellow light.

4 Another three to four minutes later, move to the fourth gate, Anahata, which is near the heart and thymus gland. This is envisaged as a green flower with 12 petals and is associated with love, compassion and nurturing. Imagine it glowing with a green light for three to four minutes.

5 The fifth gate, Vishuddi, is in the throat, near the thyroid gland. Envisage this as flower with 16 petals, glowing with a light, sky blue light. It is associated with communication, thought and speech.

6 After three or four minutes, move to the sixth Gate, Ajna, which is located at the point between the eyebrows and near the pineal gland. This is envisaged as a dark blue or indigo flower with two petals and is the location for psychic ability.

7 Having meditated for three to four minutes on the dark blue light of Ajna, move onto the final, seventh gate, Sahasrara, located at the top of the head. This is envisaged as a flower with 1,000 petals in violet or white. Sahasrara is associated with spirituality and enlightenment.

8 Now, reverse the process and step down through Ajna, Vishuddi, Anahata, Manipura, Svadhisthana and finally, to Muladhara. Spend enough time at each point to see if you can recognize any sensations in the chakras, then move onto the next one. You might like to go round the body a dozen or more times before trying the next step.

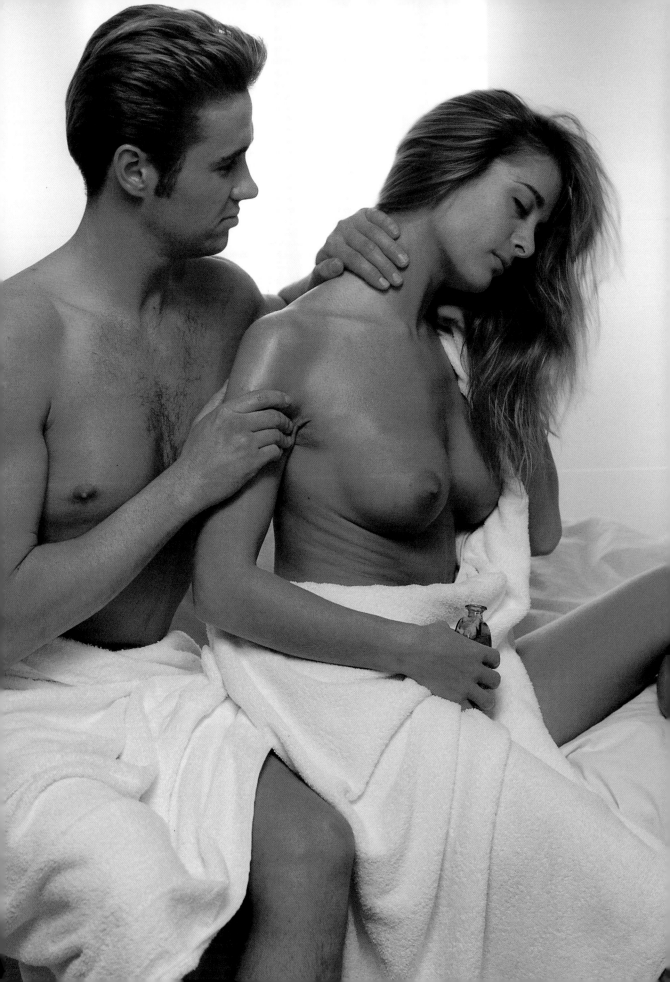

Once you have located and energized the chakras, now is the time to use them to pull energy into yourself. Visualize one of your chakras, the petalled wheel glowing with its own colour. Start with the red, four-petalled Muladhara chakra. Now breathe in and imagine the colour deepening as you inhale, glowing even brighter as you exhale. Then, think of the chakra itself as being the 'nose' that breathes in and out. As you breathe, you pull in air and direct it to your lungs to be transported in your blood to every part of your body.

Instead of air, what you are going to do is to take in energy, or 'prana', and send it through the nadis of your body. Prana is the term used to describe life force or energy. Visualize yourself pulling in prana, and that you are doing so through the gate of the chakra, located in your perineum or vagina. Focus awareness on the Muladhara chakra and 'pull' prana directly into your body as you slowly inhale. Picture the red wheel gradually deepening in colour. Then imagine exhaling, pushing the prana out through Muladhara and seeing the red gate glowing even more brightly. Move your awareness all the way up your body through Svadhisthana, Manipura, Anahata, Vishuddi to Ajna, Sahasrara, then down the chakras to Muladhara. With each visualized breath of prana, imagine the chakra you are focusing on becoming full of energy and sensation, lifting you up and making you feel rooted, creative, expressive, compassionate, communicative, in touch and enlightened.

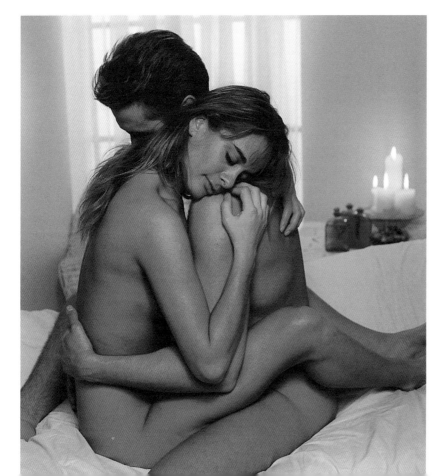

opposite: The power of touch energizes, contributing to the flow of energy between you and your partner.

left: Pass energy, or 'prana', from one to the other by aligning your chakras (see pages 16–17).

39

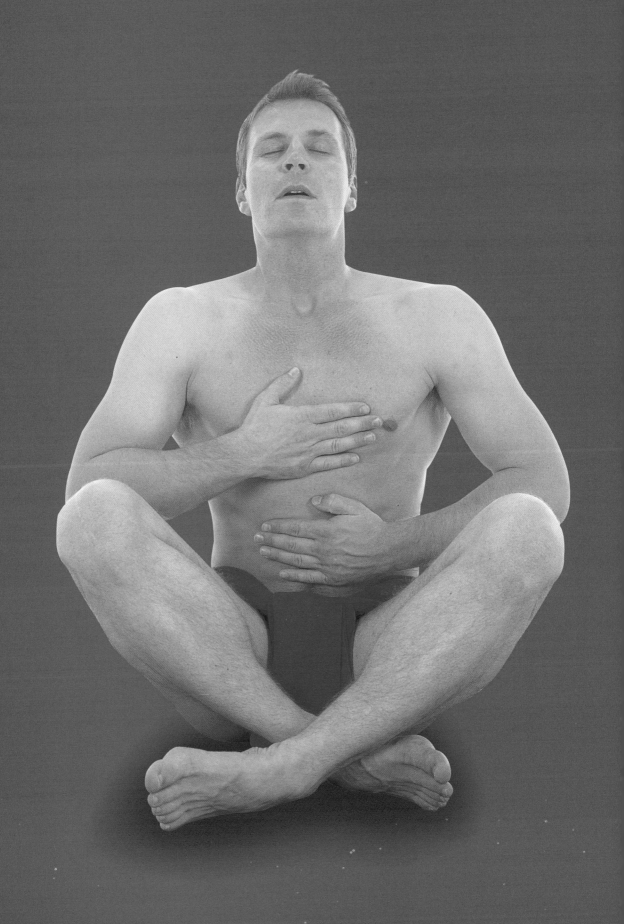

YOGA POSITIONS

As well as mantras, Tantrikas use yantras to invoke the spirit of Shiva and Shakti within themselves. The word 'yantra' means 'instrument' and yantras are the visual equivalent of mantras. They are geometric diagrams you can fix your mind upon while meditating and each chakra has its own. However, Tantrikas believe the body to be a sacred yantra, too. Since the shape a couple's bodies can take while making love may form figures similar to the yantra diagrams, some positions are particularly well suited to energizing corresponding chakras. For the same reasons, yoga poses can help you to evoke Kundalini force and encourage it to rise up in you. Yoga combines stretches and contractions, movement and breath control, strength training and cardiovascular exercise to bring body, mind and spirit into alignment. The poses may seem to be either very gentle and almost easy – or to require extraordinary flexibility. In fact, they can be energising and relaxing, and when done with a partner, can put you on the same wavelength as you mirror and follow each other's movements.

opposite: Yoga poses can encourage the Kundalini force to rise up in you. In this way, use your body as an instrument, a conduit, for the Kundalini force.

below: The half-lotus is a modified version of the classic full-lotus position.

The Lotus

When you meditate, you often take up one of the classic yoga positions, either the half-lotus or the lotus.

1   Sitting on the floor, or on a cushion or pillow, cross your legs with one foot resting on and the other foot beneath opposite thighs.
2   The full lotus needs more flexibility; to adopt this pose, place both feet so they rest on your opposite thighs.

below: The Cobra stretches out the lower back and helps to realign the body.

The Cobra

The Cobra position tones the lower back and strengthens the muscles there – making it very useful for good sex.

1   Lie flat on your stomach with the feet together and toes pointed. Place your hands, palms flat on the floor and elbows bent, under your shoulders, but keep the elbows against your body. Point your chin down towards the floor.

2   Breathe in and raise your head up from the floor. Straighten your arms, but keep the hipbones resting on the floor. Carefully arch yourself backwards and raise your chin so you look upwards.

3   While breathing out and in normally, count to ten. On the last exhale, slowly lower yourself down onto the floor again. Repeat ten times.

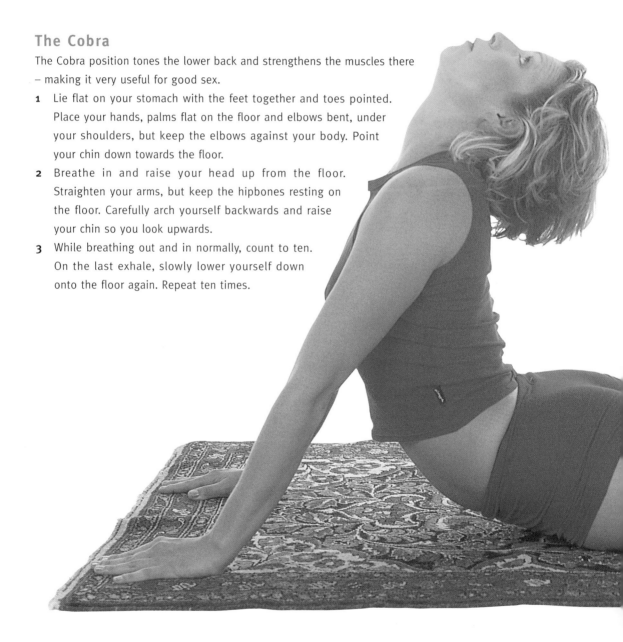

Tree Pose

This upright stance helps you to focus and concentrate.

1   Start by standing upright, with your hands by your sides, your back straight and your weight on both feet.
2   Shift your weight onto your right foot and when you have your balance, bend your left knee outwards and lift your left foot off the floor.
3   Place your left foot on your right inner thigh, as high up as you can reach and still be comfortable. Make sure your toes point down towards the floor.
4   Lift your arms up over your head and extend your fingers towards the ceiling. Breathe evenly and comfortably.
5   When you are ready to bring your foot down, take a breath; as you release it, bring your foot down and position yourself evenly on both feet in the standing pose again. Repeat on the other side, lifting the right knee.

Turned Shiva Posture

This posture helps strengthen your sense of balance and concentration, and tones the muscles of the hips, legs and chest.

1   Stand with your feet together and your arms by your sides.
2   Inhale and, as you do so, bend the left leg backward and grasp the left foot with your left hand. At the same time, extend your right arm straight out in front of you to help your balance.
3   Gradually raise your right arm upwards until it is above your head, while lifting the left leg as high behind you as you can. Hold this pose and breathe gently. To help you balance, fix your sight on something that doesn't move (i.e. not your partner!) at eye level.
4   Remain like this for about one minute, then slowly return to the standing position. Repeat on the other side, bending the right leg back and raising the left arm upwards.

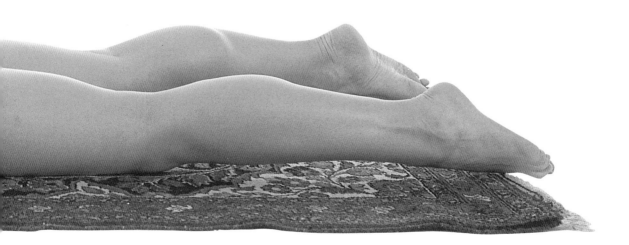

below: Prepare for sexual encounters and increase the flexibility of the spine with the Cat Stretch.

The Cat Stretch

The Cat Stretch releases tension in the spine and relieves back pain. An excellent opposite and balancing stretch to the Cobra, it is a sensuous pose, especially if you imagine yourself as the animal for which it is named.

1   Kneel on your hands and knees with your back straight. The hips should be directly above your knees and the shoulders above your hands.

2   Inhale and, as you do so, lower your head, pull in your stomach muscles and allow your back to arch up.

3   Now relax into your first position and repeat step 2. Repeat ten times.

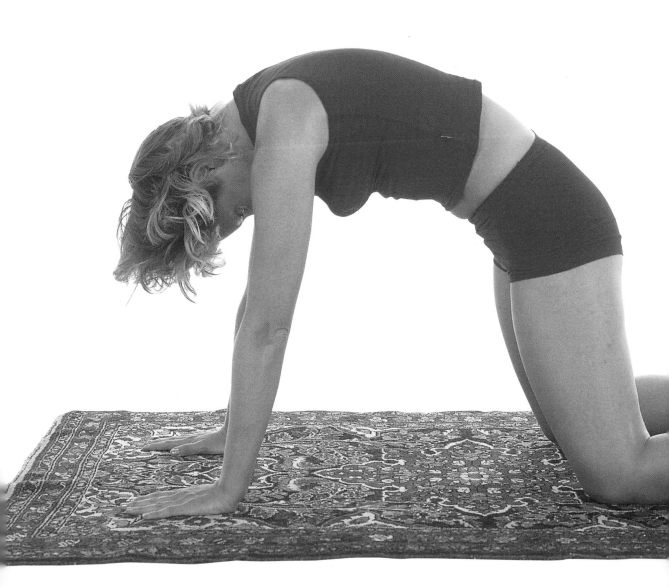

Corpse Pose

This is a relaxation pose, ideal for finishing off a yoga session.

1 Lie down flat on your back on the floor. Make sure your feet don't touch and that the toes fall outwards. Position your hands slightly away from your body, palms facing upwards and relaxed.

2 Close your eyes and breathe evenly and comfortably through your nose. Starting at your heels, imagine them becoming soft and limp, and then relaxing into the floor.

3 Move up your feet to the toes, and then up to your ankles and calves, thinking of each muscle and then letting it soften and relax as you go. Move up past your shins to your kneecaps, and the backs of the knees, to your thighs, and the backs of the thighs, and then to your hips and genitals.

4 Imagine your backside sinking into the floor. Relax the entire pelvic region. Let your attention drift up past your waist, your spine and back, your ribs and then your chest and collarbone.

5 Relax your shoulders and move down your upper arms to your elbows and forearms. Relax your wrists, palms and the backs of your hands, and then your fingers and thumbs.

6 Now relax the muscles of your neck, throat and jaw. Relax your chin and let the corners of your mouth go soft, turning them slightly upward into a hint of a smile. Flare your nostrils and relax the muscles of your cheeks, around your eyes and in your temples. Let your brow relax so all those frown lines and deep furrows disappear.

7 Finally, imagine the muscles in your scalp loosening and relaxing. Stay still for 10 minutes.

8 When you want to get up, wiggle your fingers and toes. Circle your wrists and ankles. Gently stretch your arms, legs and back.

9 Take a deep breath and pull your knees up towards your chest. With your hands behind your knees, hug them into your chest.

10 Roll over onto one side for a few minutes and then push yourself up slowly, uncurling one vertebrae at a time and letting your head come up last of all.

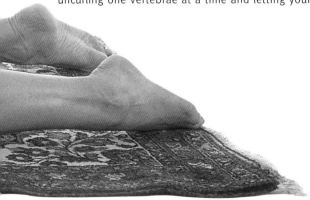

MOVEMENT

Movement and dance are important aspects of the quest for spirituality and togetherness in Tantric sex. Vatsyayana describes dance as being the third of the Sixty-four Arts. Sex itself is an intimate dance between two people that mirrors and allows them to merge with the cosmic dance. Shiva is often represented in Hindu legend as the god of dancing, the Lord of the Dance. His dance represents divine activity as the source of movement in the universe, creating and destroying, incarnating and liberating. When couples wish to identify with Shakti and Shiva in their lovemaking, they might first come together in movement. Put on some music you find appealing – rock or pop, Western, Eastern or world music; whatever gets you moving to the rhythm. At first, stand apart and then let your fingers move, then your arms, shoulders, head, hips and body. Sway to the beat to find your own rhythm. Finally, begin to move your feet and dance side to side and around each other. You don't have to be skilled at dancing – winning prizes isn't the aim here. What you are doing is finding your own feel for your body's potential and showing your partner what is on offer, and letting them show you, too. When you feel ready, and once the two of you have got the measure of each other's movement and are in tune, move into each others arms and dance together. At first, be close and sensual, not sexy. Gradually, alter your movements to become more intimate and more meaningful. You may find that dancing can be as just arousing as moving together lying down.

right: Shiva, the male force, is also the Lord of the Dance.

opposite: Dance is a sensual prelude to lovemaking.

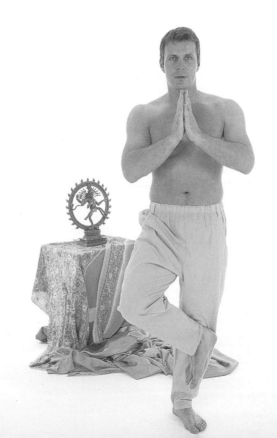

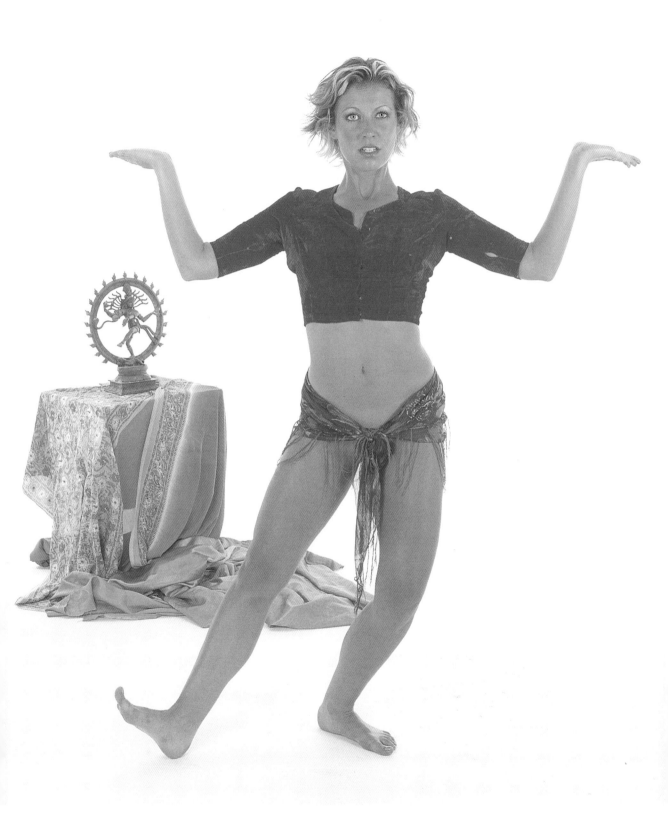

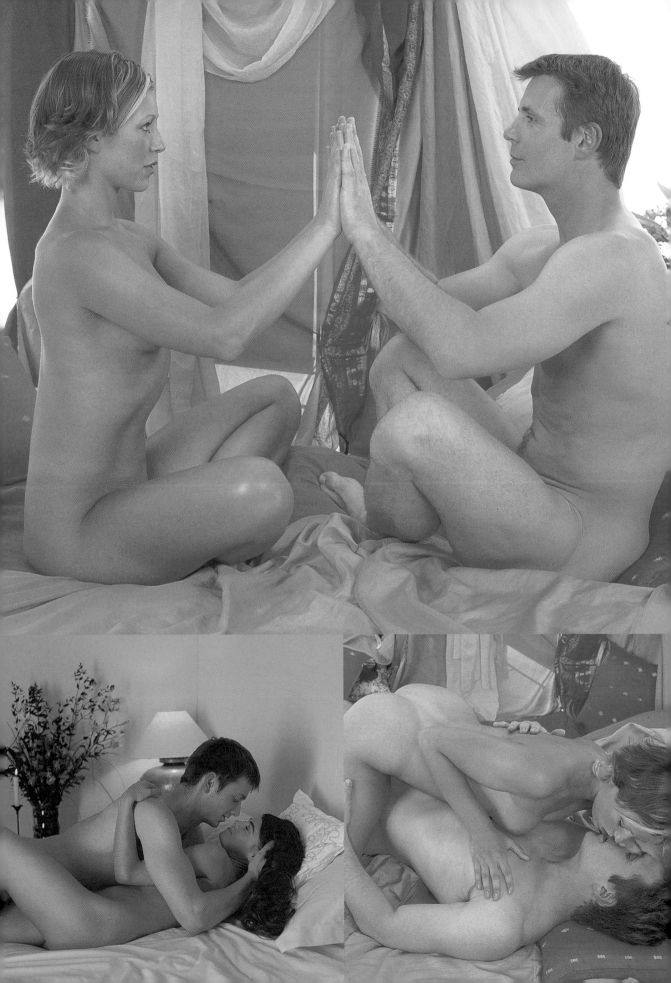

TOUCH

Touch is a particularly important sense and a vital part of your quest for enlightenment and exquisite sex. However, nonsexual touching is as significant as the sort of caresses that you would associate with romantic intimacy. The basic principles of the Tantra require that you become as accustomed to communicating and gathering information through your skin as you do through speech. You might like to try the following exercise to get in touch with your partner, and with yourself.

Sit opposite your partner, cross-legged and close to each other. Lightly stroke all the way down your partner's face, beginning above the eyes, and then stroking very gently down the cheeks, along the jawline and continuing around the neck. Stroke along the shoulders, down the arms and gently knead your partner's hands and fingers. Go back to the collarbones and brush the pads of your fingers down across your partner's chest, across the stomach, and along the thighs to the knees. Go down the shins to the feet and stroke them, then reverse the process and go back up the body, retracing your route until you get to the beginning again. Then, sit back and let your partner do the same to you. You're not trying to be sexy or arousing here, just to learn about, and get in contact with, your partner's body.

MASSAGE

Devotees of Tantric sex concentrate on the whole act of love, making foreplay and sex play before and after orgasm even more important than the orgasm itself. This approach to sex not only makes the entire experience more sensual and more exciting, but it also has the beneficial effect of prolonging both lovemaking and climax itself.

You can use massage within Tantric sex as a prelude to penetration, as foreplay, or make touching and caressing each other a pleasure in itself. Tantrikas use massage to relax and energize each other. Touching your partner's body allows you to connect with them on physical, emotional and spiritual levels. Tantrikas believe that energy flows through the body in much the same way that blood runs through veins and arteries. This energy connects the body's 'chakras,' or energy centres, most commonly thought to be at the base of the spine, the genitals, the stomach, the throat, the forehead and the crown of the head. By reaching high sexual arousal, practitioners of Tantric sex, 'open up the chakras,' or move the energy up through these physical channels to create a sensation of oneness and ecstasy. However, massage has the same effects by allowing you to come in contact with your partner's body and focus on them.

above left: Eye to eye and hand to hand begins the ritual to love.

below left: Touching allows you to communicate your inner thoughts and desires

below right: Becoming one in ecstasy, through skin-to-skin contact, takes time.

GIVING A MASSAGE

above right: Massage can involve simply stroking your partner with cream or oil.

centre: Kneading muscles takes a little know-how, but follow your partner's reactions if you are unsure.

below left: Half an hour of gentle massage puts you both in touch with your bodies.

below right: Concentrate on nonsexual areas, too, for a full-body massage.

Invite your partner to put themselves totally in your hands. Make a comfortable and safe space by spreading out a sheet, blanket or towel, with cushions or pillows for support, on the floor or another firm surface. If desired, dim lights, light candles and play quiet, relaxing music. Make sure the temperature of the room is warm, and have one or more smaller blankets or towels to hand to cover them, or parts of their body, if they become cold during the massage. Let your partner lie back and become relaxed. While lying on their back, keep a small pillow or rolled towel beneath their neck and another behind their knees. While on their front, place a rolled towel or small cushion or pillow under their shins.

Warm your hands and pour a generous handful of cream or oil into your palms. Rub them together to warm up the lotion before you begin contact with your partner's skin. Ask your partner to lie on their stomach and start with their feet and legs, moving upwards. You may want to simply stroke your partner, gently brushing them with your palms or the flats of your fingers. You can also knead muscles and gently pummel them. As you practise, you'll soon learn what touches you like and what works for your partner, too. Always begin gently, with quite broad strokes and always end by leaving your hands at rest and in contact with your partner's body for a few moments before lifting the hands away. Stroke and rub the calves and up the back of the thighs. Sweep your hands over and around the buttocks before moving up your partner's back, stroking and rubbing the small of their back, then up along their backbone to the shoulder blades. Move up to the neck and shoulders, kneading and rubbing along them. In turn, massage gently down each arm, brushing the inside of the elbows and manipulating and stroking your partner's hands and fingers.

Ask your partner to turn over on their back. Begin again at the feet and work your way up the body. Manipulate and stroke the feet, continuing up the shins, knees and thighs to the genital area. You can gently touch here, but do not make your caresses sexual. Move up your partner's stomach and chest to the collarbone and throat. Now caress your partner's face, gently stroking the jaw, the cheeks, circling the cheekbones and up to the eyebrows, and then the forehead and finally the head, massaging the scalp.

Rub, stroke and knead, listening to your partner's responses to get directions from them as to what feels good. Rest your hands on them for a moment before lifting them away, and then take a break, allowing time for your partner to rouse. Now, it's your turn to be massaged. Change places and let your partner do the same to you. It will take over half an hour, if not an hour, to massage one of you – take your time and don't hurry.

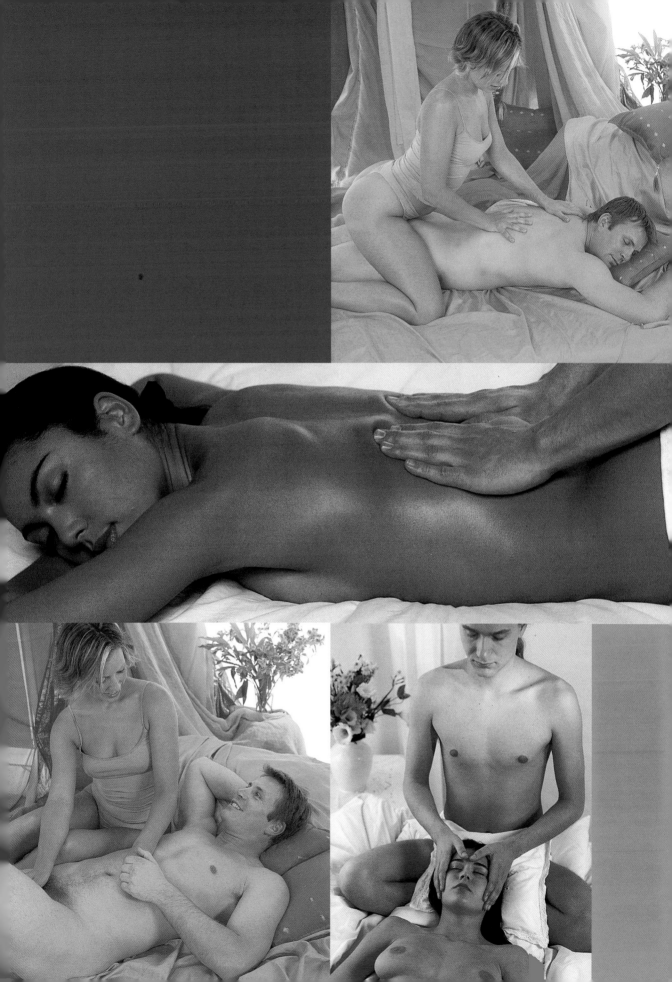

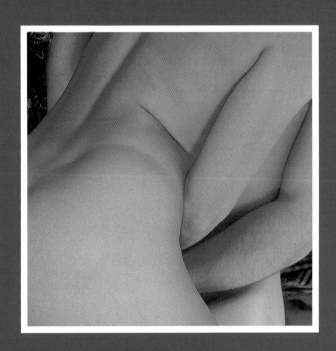

GETTING
IN TOUCH

3

TANTRIC SEX IS ALL ABOUT
LEARNING – LEARNING TO
KNOW YOURSELF. LEARNING
TO KNOW YOUR PARTNER.
SEXUAL PLEASURE ISN'T
A SUBJECT WE UNDERSTAND
INSTINCTIVELY – FIRST, WE
HAVE TO DISCOVER WHAT
PLEASES US AS WELL AS
WHAT MAY AROUSE AND
SATISFY OUR PARTNERS.

The only way you're going to learn about Tantric sex is by keeping an open mind, experimenting and experiencing and, most importantly, by communicating. The strength of Tantric sex is that it sets the scene and puts you in an atmosphere that says that sex is acceptable, that pleasure is a force for good.

Practising Tantric sex positively encourages you and your partner to discover and disclose exactly what you feel, what you need and what you like, to yourselves and to each other. To reach your true potential and discover the ways in which you and your lover can really satisfy each other, you need to open up. Within the safety of the Tantric sex ritual, you will find that easy.

Learning to love and appreciate, to know and understand yourself are essential parts of good loving. We are not born knowing how to satisfy ourselves sexually, and we need to learn this. Nor are we born equipped with the knowledge of how to please a partner. No-one can read minds and so, as well as learning about sexual pleasure, you need to know how to pass your knowledge on. There are plenty of ways of communicating, and language is not the most common or even the most effective one. What is vital, however, is to 'be in touch' with your partner, both in body and in words. Tantric sex enables and encourages you to open up the lines of communication, to build up habits of understanding and expressing between you both, becoming relaxed about being in physical contact and more comfortable with talking and sharing. The more you open up yourself to your partner and take what they tell and show you on board, the better your sex life and your relationship will be.

Sexual pleasure begins with self-knowledge. The more confident you are in knowing your own sexual responses and feelings, the easier it becomes to share this knowledge with your lover. It's a sad fact that for many of us sex is less enjoyable than we'd like or ever hoped it might be. Even when our loving relationships are going well, the sex itself may leave a lot to be desired. There are quite a few reasons for this. One may be that we tend to shy away from looking at or exploring our own bodies, convinced that they are unattractive or out of bounds. Another common reason may be that we have neither the knowledge nor the practice to know how a partner can best satisfy us or how we can please them. While the urge to have sex may be instinctive, realizing how to get the best out of lovemaking is not.

RETURN TO FIRST PRINCIPLES

To prepare yourself for pleasure, you may need, with your partner, to return to first principles. As a baby or toddler, you probably explored your own body to find out where you began and ended, and to discover what felt good and what was even better. The problem is that you probably also had your hands slapped and were told off. What this taught you was that your body was dirty, your feelings perverted and sexual exploration is a thoroughly bad thing. Left to themselves children make these discoveries as preschoolers and then put them away for future reference. Several years later, as puberty arrives, the body awakens and all those lessons are recalled and come into focus. As teenagers, most young people then resume their happy exploration of their own body, gradually doing it in the company of another young person and the two of them benefit from the lessons each have learned. Sadly, what actually tends to happen to most of us is that when our hormones start telling us that the time is ripe, what we remember from our childhood is lessons in secrecy, guilt and fear. Teenagers do explore their bodies but are often convinced they must be ugly, distasteful and not-to-be-touched. Boys masturbate but do so hurriedly and furtively in order not to be caught out – which, of course, gives them an excellent grounding in premature ejaculation. Girls may masturbate, but know they should never own up to this, or they will get a bad reputation. So it's hardly surprising that as adults many of us find it hard to appreciate, love or pleasure ourselves, and so find it just as hard to allow a partner to do so. We don't know how to give ourselves pleasure and neither does a partner.

SELF-APPRECIATION AND AFFIRMATION

Self-exploration and self-understanding are vital keys to good lovemaking within a relationship. A basic principle in Tantric sex is learning how to appreciate

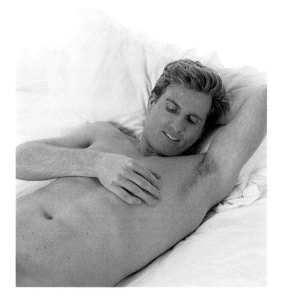

below: Tantra teaches you to know and love yourself.

yourself. It's hard for anyone to either accept or give sexual pleasure if they don't like themselves. One of the sad results of being made to feel that sensual exploration is bad is not only are you told that your sexual desires are unacceptable but that you yourself are, too. If you have been brought up to feel that you shouldn't touch yourself, you may believe that not only are your desires wrong, but your body is, too. Doctors, counsellors and agony aunts often hear from people who are convinced that their bodies are unacceptable and ugly – too fat, too thin, too tall, too short. Many of us are sure our genitals are the wrong shape, size, colour or texture; that they smell, are far too hairy or not hairy enough. In almost every case, what you have is a completely normal and perfectly acceptable body.

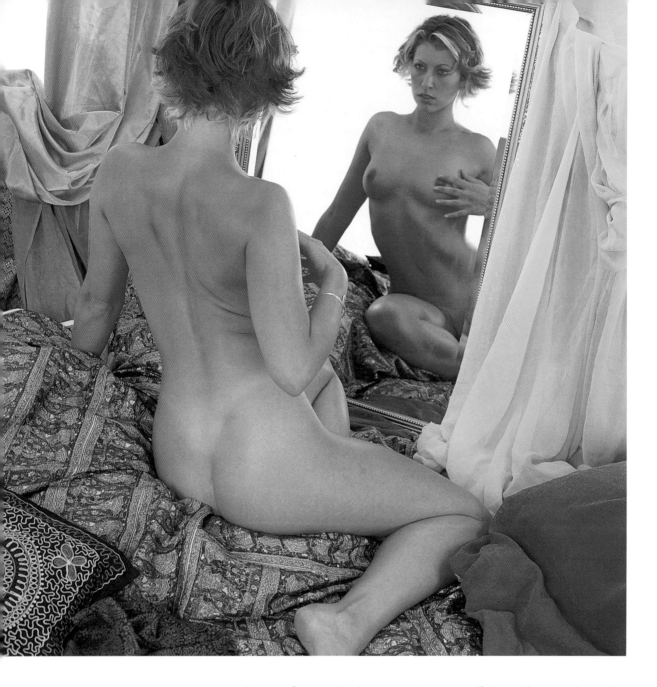

So, your first exercise is to appreciate yourself. Set aside some time to be alone and strip off, stand in front of a mirror and look at yourself. Slowly consider yourself from top to bottom and side to side. Do a slow twirl so you can see yourself all the way round. You may hear a voice in your head telling you that you are too fat or too skinny. You may feel your genitals are too small if you are a man, or too hairy if you are a woman. If you are a woman, you may think your breasts are too big, too small, too droopy or with too many stretchmarks. You may think you haven't enough muscles or hair – or are too hairy on your body with not enough on top of your head, if you are a man.

Now take another look at yourself. This time, banish any negative voices and listen for the ones that are positive. With fresh eyes, start thinking about what someone who loved you would see. Begin thinking about what you would see, if you hadn't been told or taught, or picked up all those reservations about your own body. You are gorgeous, whatever your shape or size, and it's time to realize that. Look at yourself and pick one part that you like, and tell yourself, 'you have great eyes/hair/toes'. Say it again, and promise yourself you will repeat this to yourself from now on, at least once a day. Each day, find another part of you that you realize is attractive, and add it to the list.

Next, close your eyes. Slowly and carefully run your hands all over your body, gently feeling and experiencing yourself. Notice the different textures of your skin, depending on whether it's the skin on your face or the back of your hands, the soles of your feet or the inside of your thighs that you're touching. Focus on the palms of your hands. Are they rough and calloused, or soft and smooth? Which texture would feel better on what part of your body? Open your eyes and repeat the procedure again, watching your hands and each part of your body as you touch and explore.

FOCUSED EXPLORATION

Now it's time to move on to some more focused exploration. For this, you might like to sit or lie down. Make sure you are warm and comfortable. It helps, for instance, to have some cream or oil on hand, or even to do this in a warm bath with plenty of bath oil or gel in the water. Again, run your hands slowly over yourself from top to bottom, side to side and all around. Concentrate on what seems especially pleasant. You may be surprised at what simply feels good – similar to the pleasure a cat or dog may feel at being stroked. Whether we are animals or humans, all of us love the power of touch. There is nothing quite as comforting and affirming as being stroked. Smooth your hands over the fur of a cat and it will purr. Try it on your own body and allow yourself to see why the animal makes that noise. Focus, and you'll soon find that there isn't a part of your body that you can't appreciate being touched.

Once you've sensitized yourself and brought yourself alive by stroking yourself, you can concentrate on discovering the next level. This is to find and bring to life the parts of your body that tingle not only with sensual pleasure but also respond with sexual arousal to your caresses. There are obvious places – the nipples of both sexes, the clitoris and the penis. Perhaps you won't be surprised to discover that the lips are also intensely sensitive and most of us know that earlobes react strongly when they are stimulated. You wouldn't be amazed to find that the labia and the scrotum are intensely sensitive or that sucking, blowing on or nibbling toes and fingers is more than pleasant. Most people notice their necks are extremely sensitive as are the inside of your elbows and thighs and the backs of your knees. But you may find the buttocks

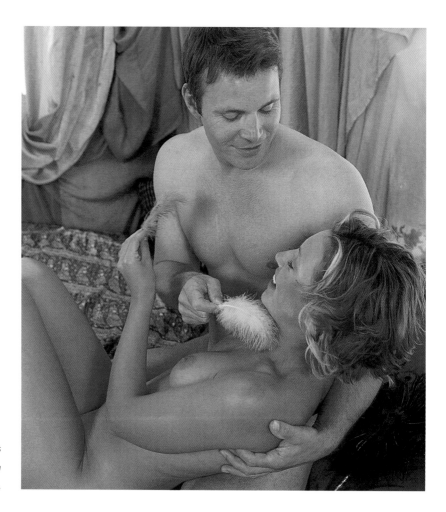

*right: Explore layers
of texture, sensation
and reaction.*

or small of the back, around the anus and down the inside of the thighs are
also very sensitive areas. You may also discover that the way you stimulate
a particular part of the body has a bearing on how it may or may not arouse
you. Stroke and tickle and experiment with different levels of touching to see
what sort of effect they have. Brush lightly with the tips or flats of your fingers
or scratch gently with your nails. Tickle or rub lightly or more firmly. You can use
the heels of your hands to massage rhythmically or press and knead with your
thumbs. Use the palms or the whole of your hand to stroke or brush large areas
of your body or concentrate on just one bit. Find those parts of yourself that
particularly please or arouse you when stimulated. Experiment with the various
caresses that really excite you.

Sensation and reaction

When you've found what gives you delight, it's time to move on to discovering
how you can really please yourself, from arousal to full satisfaction. Concentrate

on those areas that particularly excite you, but try not to stimulate only the most obvious bits. Predictably, you bring yourself to orgasm by stimulating your penis or clitoris, but both arousal and climax will be more exciting and satisfying if you stimulate as much as your body as possible, rather than just going for the main area. Take your time, and use your fingers and anything else that comes to hand to build up layers of sensation and reaction.

Self-pleasuring can be all the more satisfying if you introduce different ways of fondling yourself – strokes, caresses, nips, pinches, scratches and even smacks. It can also be better if you introduce contrasting textures. Pour some oil or cream all over yourself and see how it feels to glide and squidge your hands across your body. Use a feather to tease and tweak and touch, or try some fake fur, a silk scarf or a scratchy facecloth or towel. See the difference if you dip a sponge first into hot water, then into cold, before wiping it over the sensitive parts of your body. There is no rush, so pursue every last scrap of enjoyment. Pay special attention to anything that seems to set your teeth on edge or make you jump – pain or discomfort is often the other side of the coin of pleasure. If at first it makes you shy away, it could in fact be the touch that is going to give you the greatest result. Bring yourself to full arousal and continue until you've come to an orgasm. And do not stop there. Both sexes find being hugged and held particularly comforting after orgasm, so lie down, snuggle up and hug yourself to complete the pleasure. You are likely to enjoy the sensation of rhythmic stroking on your arms, face and back for some time after orgasm. And indeed, for some people, it need not stop with your first orgasm. The vast majority of women are capable of more than one, and often several, orgasms at a time. Continue to explore your sensations after you have come and you may find the next climax is even better than the first. Some men, too, discover a potential for multiple orgasms at this stage, although we will explore how many if not most men can become multi-orgasmic later on.

SHARING

Once you have had a chance to appreciate yourself and your body, and to explore your reactions and responses on your own, it's time to share those discoveries with your partner. Set aside a time when you and your partner can spend several hours on your own together with no interruptions. Stand in front of the mirror again but this time with your partner. Practise being at ease with standing in some light, naked, and looking at yourself and them. Tell them what you see in yourself and discuss the bits you like and dislike and why. Ask them which parts of you they find attractive, and look at that part of your body with a new appreciation. You may be surprised, because they may find attractive or even arousing a bit you can't stand. Trust and believe your partner, and do the same for them.

EXPLORING EACH OTHER

Sit down in comfort with your partner, with perhaps one of you leaning back against your partner's knees or into their lap. Take the time to look at and stroke each other's bodies, telling and showing your partner the bits you like, the ones you want to touch and adore. At this stage, avoid touching the more sexual areas – the genitals and the breasts. Concentrate on every other part of the body, from toes to fingers to the crown of the head. Caress and make much of each other, using combs and hair brushes for their hair, emery boards to touch up their nails, lotion or cream to pamper their hands, arms, back or stomach. Make a point of exploring touch, taste, smell and sound on your own and your partner's body: the texture and taste of it, the smell and the sound made when you stroke or scratch it. Bring your senses alive by sharing scents and tastes you both enjoy, such as flowers, incense, favourite foods or drink, as you relax and get to know each other in this way. Cosset each other in every way you can imagine until you both feel truly valued and loved.

below: Truly look at your partner, and tell them what feels good.

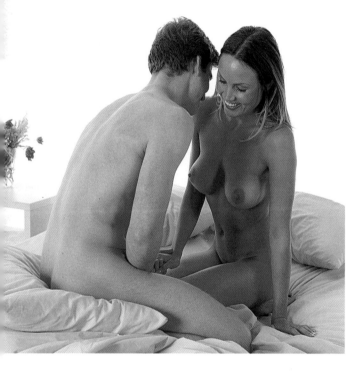

Sexual touching

Now kneel down, face to face, with your partner. Touch and caress each other, starting with hands and moving up the arms to the shoulders, around the neck and down the torso. Turn and turn about, demonstrate to your partner what you've found in your sessions of self exploration. Touch your own body, and guide their hands, talking your partner through how various caresses on different places feel. Experiment with different touches and textures. Use your nails to gently scratch your partner, trailing your nails down their chest or back, or up their legs or arms. Use gentle scratches or harder ones, always asking them whether it feels good or not and acting accordingly. Rub with the flats of your fingers or knead harder with the fingertips or knuckles. Sweep a feather or a loofah, or a sponge or nail brush, over their body to arouse them.

opposite top: Explore taste sensations as well as touch to evoke passion.

opposite centre: Guide each other's hands to the places that feel nice.

opposite below: Stimulate with scents and scratches to find pleasure points.

Use your tongue, lips and teeth to lick, suck, nibble and gently bite your partner. Find out from their response what feels good, what they find discomforting and what is positively arousing. Pay special attention to the specific areas of the body (see the following tips, pages 62–4), using your hands and mouth to stimulate every inch of your partner's body.

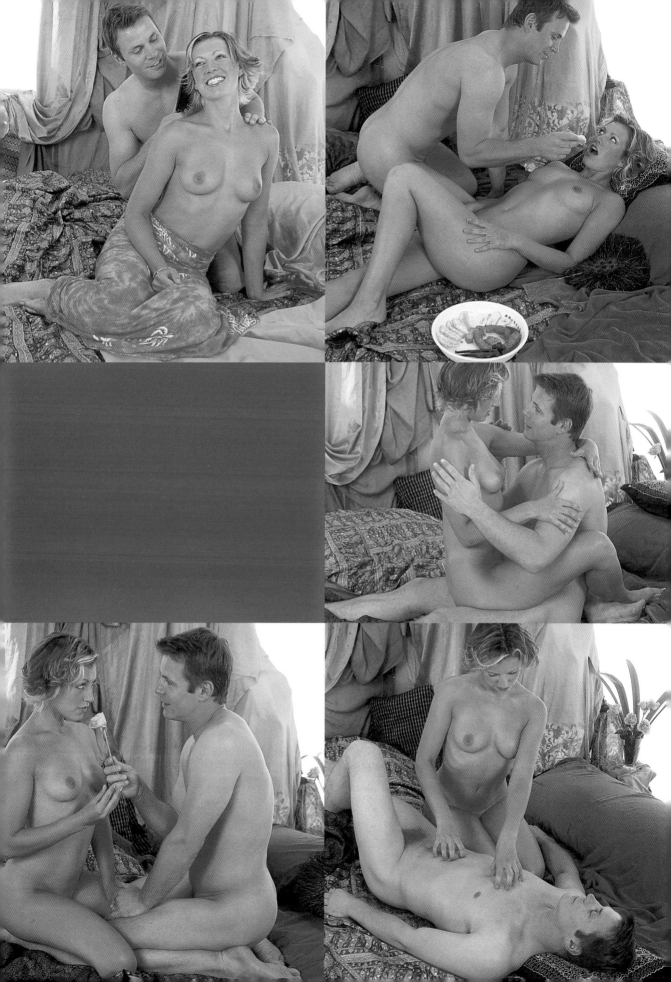

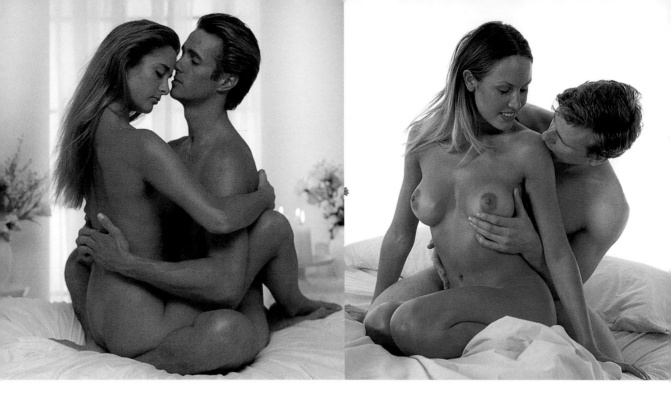

- Caress your partner's face, from above the eyebrows, down the nose, up over the cheekbones and down the jawline to the chin. Gently extend the caresses down to the neck, chest, stomach and the genitals. Use your fingertips and only brush lightly. Bring the caress back up again to the nose. This creates a circle of energy, which encompasses your partner from nose to lingam or yoni. The tip of the nose is on a central line or meridian, which connects the nose right down to the Muladhara, or root, chakra. Touching it sends energy flowing through that meridian. When you trace the meridian with your fingertips down to the root chakra and then up again to the nose, you create a complete circuit of energy which awakens your partner's sexual desires.

- Gently manipulate the area where the shoulders join the neck. You can nibble, suck or bite, scratch, squeeze or press. Using your thumbs, carefully knead and massage up the back of the neck to the base of the skull. This releases a lot of the tension carried in the shoulders and neck. The neck is also on the line that connects directly to the lower back and the pelvis – two key areas for sexual feelings. As stress tension here recedes, sexual tension will rise up.

- Take your partner's hand in yours and gently locate the crease of the wrist, the point where the hand and wrist join. Caress, lick and kiss this area, warming it with your breath. This transmits energy to the heart and to the fourth chakra, Anahata, the centre of desire, affection and love.

- Very gently massage either side of the throat, just behind the jawbone and a couple of inches down from the earlobe, with your fingertips. This is the site of the thyroid glands and the fifth chakra, Vishuddi. Stimulating this area is relaxing and energizing, and increases sexual response.

- Face each other and, reaching behind your partner's back, lightly rub between the shoulder blades with your palms. Gradually move closer until your upper bodies are pressed close together. Now, increase the pressure until you are massaging strongly, pressed chest to chest in each other's arms. Your hands will create energy while the close, chakra to chakra, contact of your bodies opens the gates and passes energy between you.

- Face your partner, sitting in each other's laps. Take it in turns to tickle, tease, caress, nibble and kiss your partner's nipples. The nipples directly connect to the genitals and both sexes find this immensely arousing.
- Face your partner while kneeling, or let them lie down full length. Place your hand on their belly, a few inches above the pubic bone, and let your hand rest there. Imagine energy flowing from your hand into their body, through the second chakra, Svadhisthana. Stimulating this area is sensual and exciting.

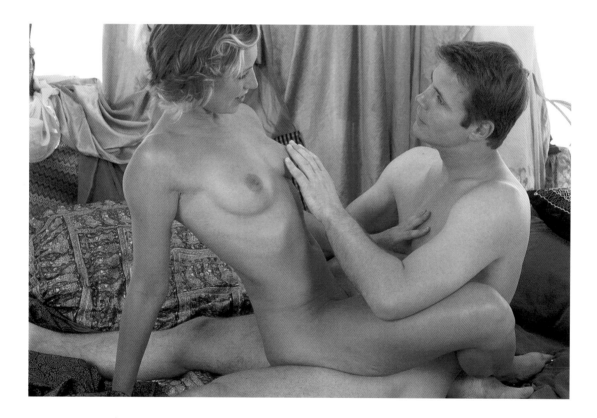

- Ask your partner to lie face down, or sit with their back turned to you. Gently at first but then more strongly, rub, massage, stroke and scratch the area above the buttocks, in the small of the back. This also stimulates the second chakra, Svadhisthana, leading to arousal and excitement.
- Ask your partner to lie down or sit, cross-legged, while you sit in their lap. Gently massage the genitals, the outside of the labia or lips (if your partner

above: The nipples are a sensitive area for both sexes.

is female), the scrotum (if male). Slowly tease and caress the skin and then gently stroke down to the inside of the groin and thigh on one side and back up on the other side to create a circuit from genitals to thighs and back. Making an energy circuit moves energy around the pelvis.

- Place one hand on your partner's yoni or lingam, and the other hand on their heart. Visualize the energy coming from the heart, the place of passion and love, and imagine it flowing through you to their genitals, the place of pleasure.

- Take one of your partner's feet in your hands. Kiss and caress it, taking special care of the toes. Sucking toes and licking in between them drains tension and invites relaxation. For some people, it can be very arousing, to the point of climax. The hollow between the Achilles tendon and the ankle bone is on the line that goes to the kidneys. Massaging here is reputed to stimulate sexual arousal.

below: Imagine energy flowing from the heart to the genitals.

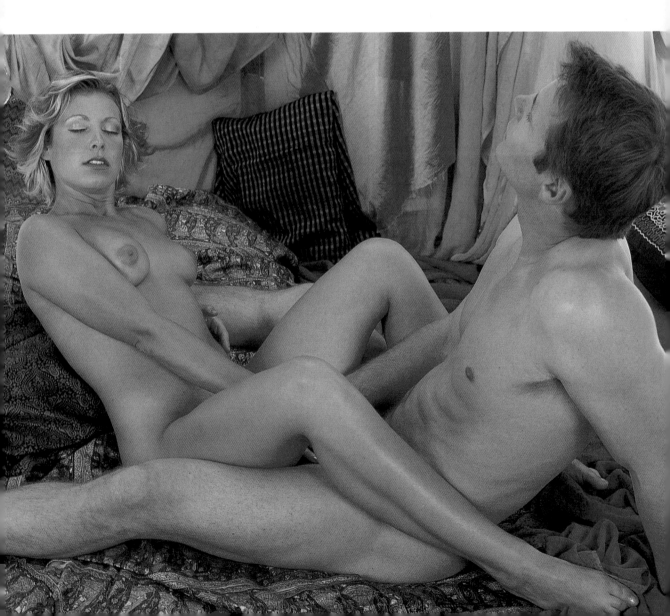

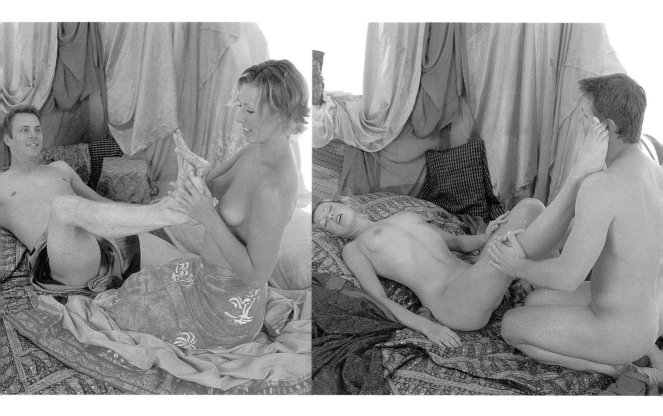

COMMUNICATING

What you are aiming to do is twofold: to find out what pleases you and what pleases your partner. The other, equally important aspect, is to learn how to let your partner know what you are thinking and feeling by telling them. You can do this in words, or by sighing or relaxing. The only important thing to remember is that your partner can't read your mind. For both of you to get in touch, you need to communicate. And, of course, they are going to have to let you know their response, so listening with your whole body as well as your ears is vitally important. If you're not sure, ask each other and check it out.

Above all, take your time. What makes lovemaking so disappointing so many times, for so many people, is that they tend to rush straight onto the main action. When we talk about making love or having sex, what usually comes to mind is full-on intercourse and orgasm. The 'Big O' is usually seen as the point of erotic activity and it's often the only part we consider or value. What Tantric sex is all about is that plus everything else – and often, the 'everything else' aspect becomes as pleasurable and satisfying, if not far more, than the climax itself. The longer you take to build up to the climax, the more you not only enjoy the ending but also the getting there. So, just as you did for yourself,

above left: Massaging feet can bring on arousal and even orgasm.

above right: Sighs and groans tell you what you want to hear.

lie back with your partner and start by running your hands all over each other's bodies. As with yourself, use the tips and flats of your fingers, the palms and the whole of your hands, and vary your strokes from feather touches, scratches and nips to kneads and light slaps. Feel and probe and tell each other how much pleasure you are getting from touching them and listen out for what they can tell you about how they are receiving your ministrations.

Triggers of arousal and stimulation

Once you have acquainted yourself with your partner's entire body and they have with yours, focus more intently on what arouses and stimulates you both. This is where you need to direct your partner to the parts of your body that are especially responsive and to let them do the same for you. Keep in mind each other's individuality. What works for one of you may not be the same for the other. In fact, what drives you wild might leave your partner cold or even irritated. Just because something gives you specific pleasure, don't assume you should try it out on them or that they will like it. Allow your partner to help you to explore and learn what really pleases them, and let them learn what pleases you, too. While men and women have many similarities in tastes and their physiology, there are also some particular differences that you need to be aware of. A man's climax is delightfully and easily achieved simply by stimulating

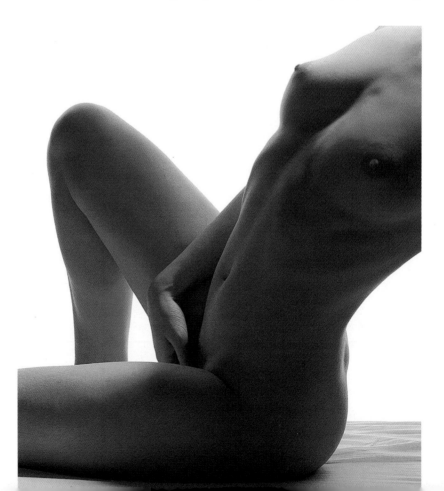

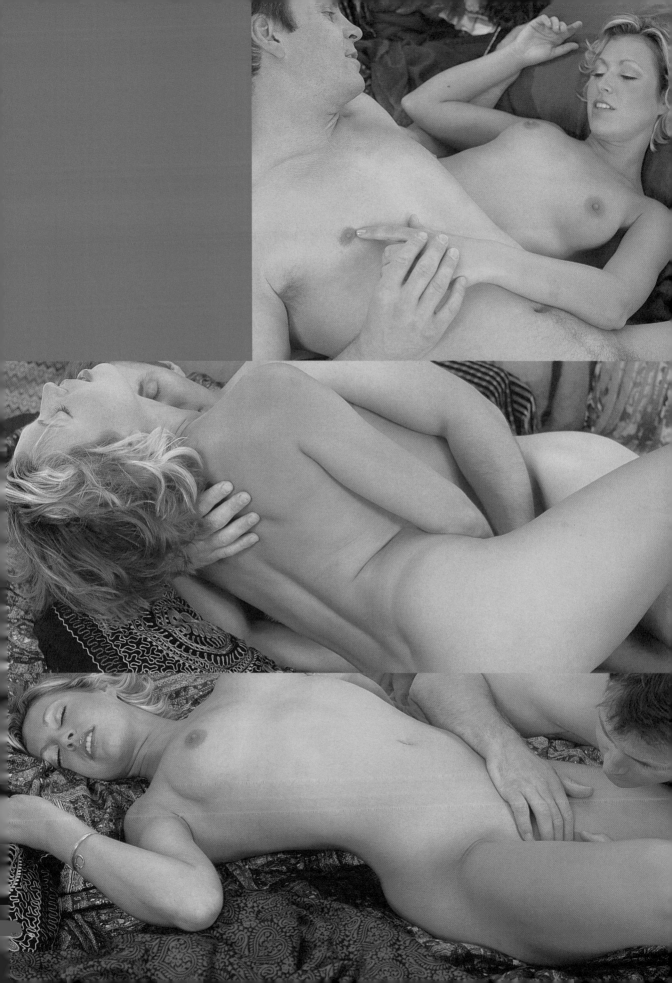

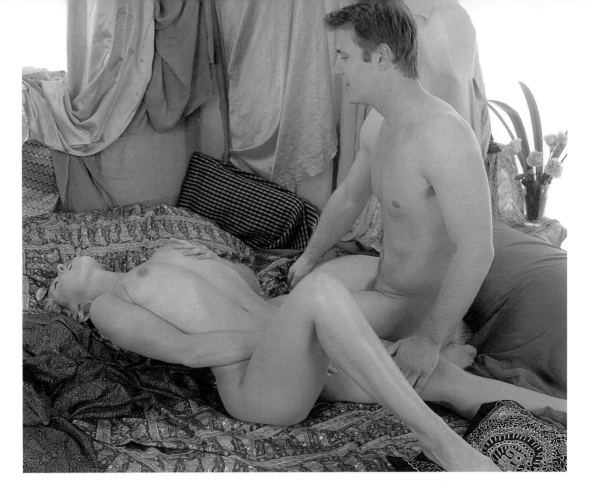

above: *For a man, watching his partner pleasure herself is arousing and educational.*

his penis, either by enfolding it in the snug, warm embrace of a vagina or a hand. This has led many people to assume vaginal intercourse is also the best way for women to climax. For a woman to have an orgasm, however, she needs her clitoris to be stimulated and this isn't always best done through intercourse. It is true that the network of nerves connected to the clitoris sweep back an extraordinary long way from that small organ sited above and in front of the urethra or water passage. The clitoris has been estimated as having an area of sensitivity some 30 times larger, size for size, than a penis. This means that even during vaginal penetration the movements in this area are transmitted to the clitoris, often directly leading to orgasm.

However, many women find they prefer more direct stimulation. Either they want to have their clitoris directly touched by their own or their partner's fingers, or for different sexual positions to allow stimulation in other ways. But in many cases, what makes a woman really enjoy sex is for there to be stimulation – direct and indirect – to the clitoris, both before and after intercourse, and for penetrative sex not to be the be-all and end-all of the act. When you are both relaxed and ready, you can move onto really focusing on sexual arousal. However, you can still take your time. Just as too many lovers dash on to trying sexual arousal before they have fully explored sensual stimulation, so too do many people leap straight into penetrative sex before they have had time to explore the power of arousal without intercourse.

THE SEXUAL RESPONSE CYCLE

Taking your time when you get together allows you and your partner to be on the same wavelength when it comes to communication. It also helps you be in synch with your sexual response. Understanding the sexual response cycle can help you recognize why it is so important to be in tune when you want to set the scene for a sexual encounter with your partner. When we get aroused and go on to experience orgasm, we go through four distinct stages that are known as the sexual response cycle.

The first stage is the arousal or excitement phase. This can be triggered by thinking about sex or through seeing or hearing something you find arousing, such as a sexy image, person or situation. Or it can be begun by someone touching you, or making a sexual suggestion. During arousal, both men and women go through a series of physical changes. Men experience an erection, not only of the penis, but sometimes of the nipples. Women, too, will find both their nipples and their clitoris are likely to swell, as does the labia or area around the vagina. They'll also experience some moisture in the vagina as a prelude to sex. How long you stay in the arousal stage can vary – it can last as long as you want, or you can hurry through it in minutes if you prefer.

Arousal is followed by the second phase, the plateau stage. Plateau is a bit like that moment on a roller coaster when you reach the top of the first big drop. It's the point during which you catch a breath because you know, any moment now, you're going to need it. During plateau, both men and women will flush, not just on their faces but also on the chest, stomach, shoulders and arms. It's why women put on blusher to appear attractive and why that 'just out of the gym or off the track' sweaty look is such a turn-on. There is nothing quite as attractive as someone who looks as if they're hot and bothered at the sight of you. Both men and women will find the sexual parts of their bodies will increase in size – not just nipples and penis, but also breasts and testicles. Your blood pressure will have increased and reached quite a high rate, and your pulse will be racing and you'll be breathing fast.

Once you reach the plateau stage, you know, barring a halt in the proceedings, that the third stage, orgasm, is only 30 seconds to 3 minutes away. When the point of orgasmic inevitability is reached, it happens and nothing you can do can stop it. During orgasm, you will be panting and your heart will be pounding. Your body will also be overtaken with a series of muscular contractions that you won't be able to control.

Following orgasm is the fourth stage, resolution, during which all the changes that have happened return to normal in reverse order. The flush that has spread across your body recedes, the swollen and enlarged areas of your body decrease again, and your breathing and heart rate go back to normal.

Being in tune

The sexual response cycle is the same in men and women, and the same each
time you make love. What you actually feel and how far along the cycle you
proceed, and how quickly, may alter each time, however. Arousal, as mentioned,
can last anything from several hours to a few minutes. You can interrupt or hold
yourself back at the plateau stage, and so never reach orgasm. And, having
experienced orgasm, you can go onto another plateau and further orgasms
before reaching resolution. But the important element to concentrate on here is
the role of arousal in lovemaking. If one of you is well into being excited by the
time you and your partner start making love, or is someone who can and does
move swiftly on through the arousal stage, this time or every time, one of
you may be left trailing well behind the other. And if, as so many people
do, you jump immediately into having penetrative sex, and then roll over and
go back to sleep afterwards, it's hardly surprising if your partner is left largely
dissatisfied. It's not that one of you is slow or frigid; it's because one of you
stole a march and never let the other catch up.

So, that's why it's so important to let each other know what you're thinking,
what you're wanting and how, and when and where you would like to get it on.
And that is the tremendous promise of Tantric sex, that it encourages and helps
both partners to slow down and be in tune whenever you make love. The aim is
to either match your patterns so that both of you are at roughly the same stage
of arousal, can both be at plateau and then move on to orgasm together. Or
that one of you can linger in the arousal stage, which you can prolong for a
considerable time, until the other catches up. Or one of you, having gone
through plateau to orgasm, can then concentrate on your partner until they too
reach their end point. Better still, Tantric sex can help both of you – men

below: Take turns to bring
yourself to climax while your
partner watches. They can
then put what they've learned
from you into practise.

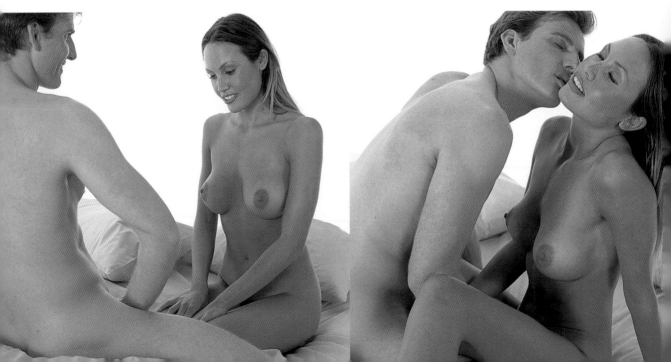

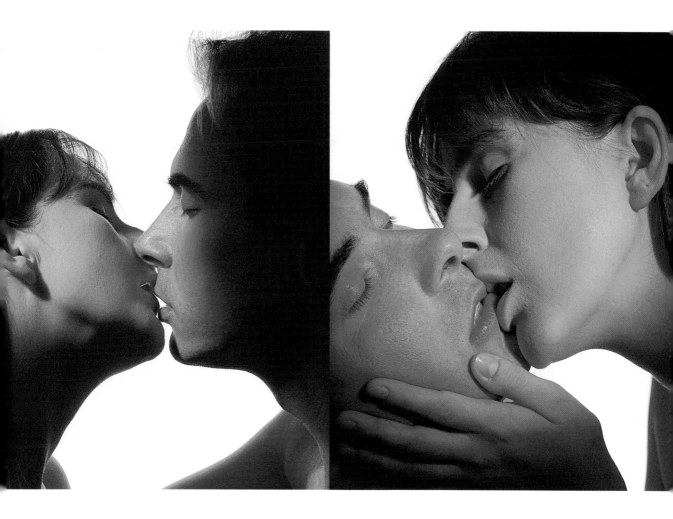

included – to enjoy more than one orgasm, or to delay orgasm and enjoy lovemaking long enough to really satisfy your partner and yourself. Even when both of you have had an orgasm, it does not need to be the end point at all. It's not just that both of you may find a capacity for more than one orgasm, there is also the fact that many people enjoy slow and gentle caresses even more after they've had an orgasm, and sexual feelings can linger long after climax. The more prepared you are, the more both of you are going to enjoy sex.

Bring yourself to arousal and then to climax as your partner watches. You could do this simultaneously, with both of you sharing by each doing the same to yourselves. But what often happens then is that you get caught up in your own sensations and forget to notice what is going on with your partner. So you may like to take turn by turn, first watching as your partner comes to a climax and then following suit with your own orgasm. Do this together a few times before moving onto the next stage, which is where you each put what you've learned from watching each other into practice.

above: Your lips are the most sensitive area, so take your time to find the kisses that turn you on most.

overleaf: Combine deep, thrusting kisses with softer more gentle ones to work up an orgasmic rhythm.

Kissing

Kissing may be thought to be a tame occupation and just a prelude to sex, but in some societies, it is considered to be the most intimate and exciting contact possible between two people. You can bring your partner, and yourself, to a climax simply by touching mouth to mouth. Tantric belief has it that there is a direct link from the upper lip – specifically, from the frenulum, which is the connective tissue inside your mouth between your upper lip and gums – to the clitoris and glans.

Start by placing light, feathery kisses all over your partner's lips. Very gently, nibble and nip their lips and around their mouth. Let the tip of your tongue stroke just inside their mouth initially, and then probe deeper, caressing inside the lips and cheeks. Thrust more firmly inside your partner's mouth, copying the thrusts the lingam (penis) may make inside the yoni (vagina). Pause every now and then to gaze into each other's eyes before continuing with your sensual kisses. See how aroused and satisfied you can get yourself and your partner simply through mouth-to-mouth contact.

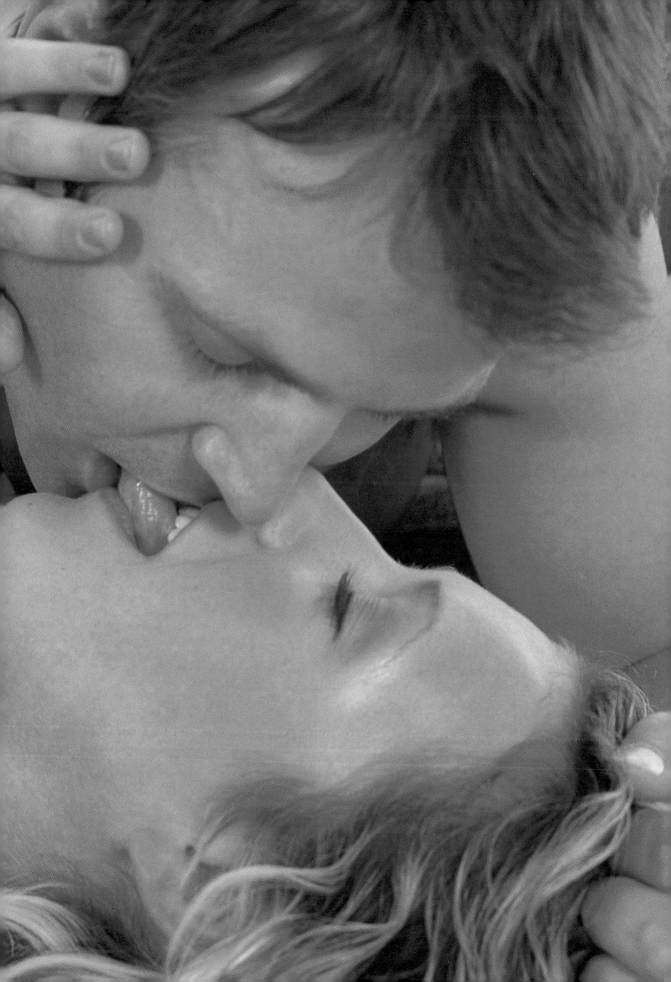

SENSATE FOCUS

To really get the benefit of exploring and getting to know your own and your partner's body and reactions you could, at this point, move into sensate focus – a way of really concentrating on the pleasure each of you may give to, and get from, each other but without the pressure of having to 'perform'. Performance fears can often spoil lovemaking for couples. The man may feel under pressure to hold himself back and move the woman along towards orgasm, while she may feel the strain of needing to 'come' during intercourse. Both of you may be intimidated by a simultaneous need to please your partner and be satisfied yourself.

One way of lifting the strain is to ban penetrative sex altogether for a while. Agree between yourselves that for a time – maybe a month or a set number of times you have sex together – you won't have intercourse at all. Instead, you and your partner can make love by enjoying caresses and any other form of arousal. Prolong your enjoyment as much as possible. Once you deny yourself the accustomed quick and easy release of penetrative sex, you will often find new ways of pleasing and being pleased. You will often discover that the pleasure you can give each other can certainly last longer, and may be better, when using hands, lips, tongues, feathers and anything else that comes to reach instead of your genitals. Try it that way for several sessions before you reintroduce intercourse.

Soul-gazing

This technique involves gazing steadily into your partner's eyes, without touching each other at all. To do this, sit cross-legged or kneel in front of each other and look long and longingly at each other. You may have a fit of the giggles the first time you try this. Persist because you may soon find that soul-gazing transmits a huge amount of sexual energy whenever you look at, and know that you have a hunger for, each other. Some couples say they can have orgasms just by gazing at each other.

Caressing

Move on to touching each other, at first only allowing yourselves caresses on parts of the body you don't normally think of as sexy – elbows, the small of the back, necks and fingers and toes. You may find touches in these areas, especially if you avoid the genitals and nipples, have as dramatic an effect as caressing the breasts, clitoris and penis. After some time avoiding the genitals, allow yourself to touch them, too. You will find that focusing your attention on all parts of the body, not just the more obvious ones, allows you to bring all of yourself and your partner to tingling arousal.

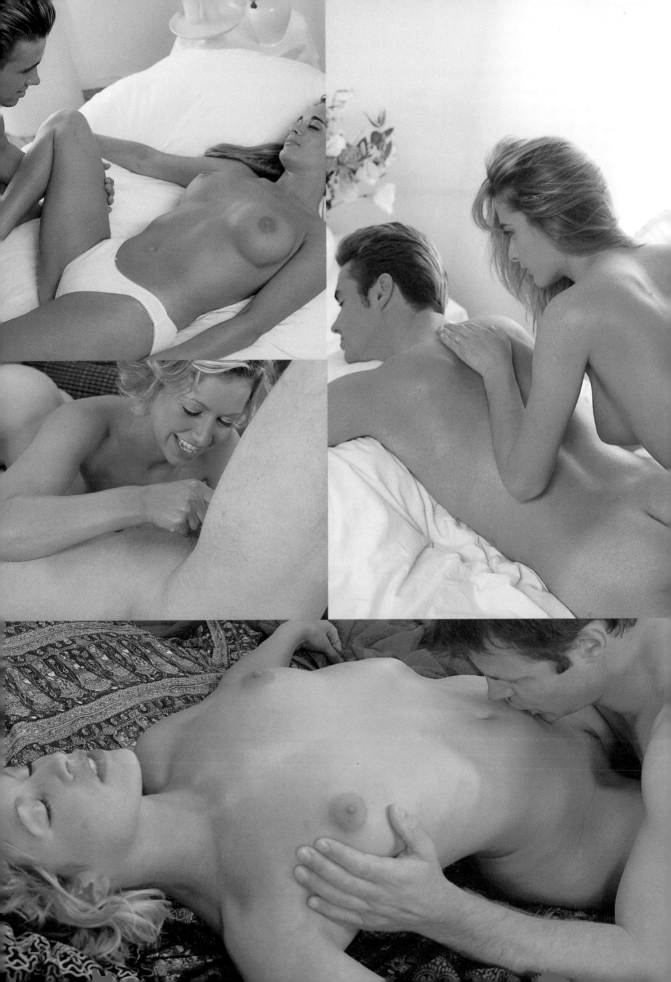

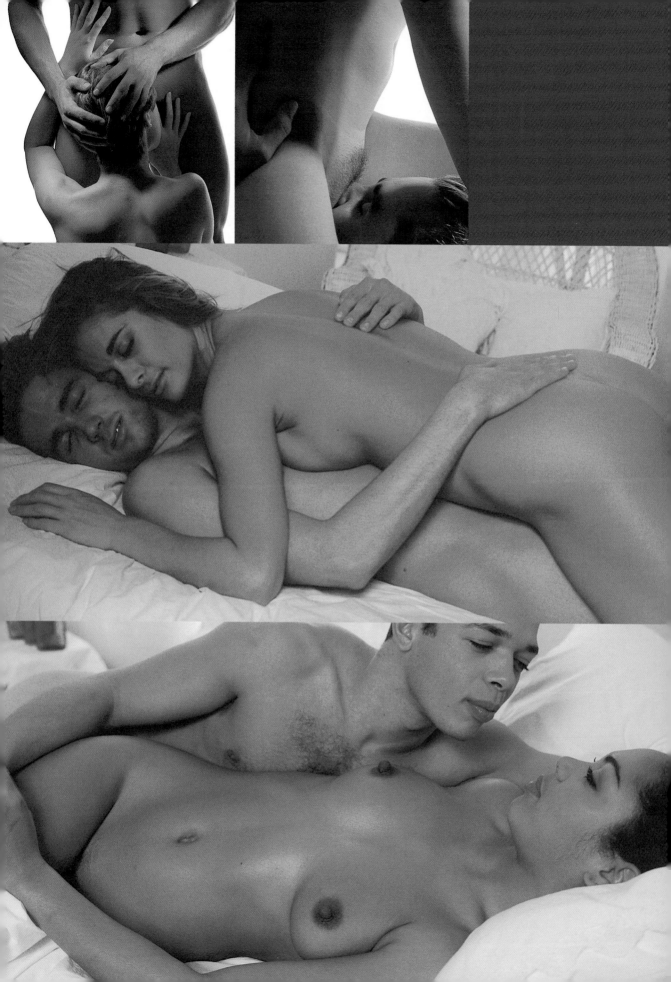

You could go one step further and try 'Look Ma, no Hands!' sex. With this technique, not only is penetrative sex banned, but so too is using hands and fingers. You can apply tongues, lips and teeth, or employ feathers, fur, silk or velvet fabrics, oil or lotion, or anything else that will stimulate your enjoyment – as long as you don't use your hands for contact. By experimenting and using your ingenuity, you will make intercourse just one of many ways to please each other, instead of one and only one.

DELAYING CLIMAXES

Tantric sex encourages the female member of a partnership to come to a climax as often as she likes and chooses. Most women are only too happy to go on to further lovemaking and find little difficulty in having multiple orgasms. But you may both find yourselves feeling some disappointment if the man comes too soon, resulting with the encounter ending before you would like. A couple can, indeed, go on 'making love' even after the man has come. You don't need an erect penis or penetrative sex for both of you to gain enjoyment and satisfaction out of a sensual encounter. Because Tantric belief places great value on men being able to continue to have penetrative sex for some time, you may like to take this opportunity to learn how the man can delay his climax and so go on to even bigger, better orgasms.

The 'Squeeze Technique'

If the man finds himself approaching the point of no return – the point at which orgasm becomes inevitable – too soon, he can stop action and wait for the feelings of excitement to recede. Sometimes this is difficult to do and he may miss the critical moment. So instead, you can make use of the 'squeeze technique'. This was a strategy first described by the sex researchers and therapists Masters and Johnson.

Either of you can perform the technique, but it works best if the woman does it. Take the man's penis in your hand, with your fingers along the top of the shaft, close to his body. Put the flat of your thumb just under the head of the penis, the glans, where the bridge of skin joins the bulbous head to the shaft. As he approaches the urgent point of no return, press firmly but gently with your thumb. The urge to come will subside and he will go a little soft, but will maintain his erection. The woman can continue stimulating him until he reaches the same point, when the technique can be repeated as many times as you both can stand it. When the man becomes better at controlling himself, the woman can also apply the 'squeeze technique' while he is inside her by pressing at the base of the penis. Then take a break, lie back and relax together before once again moving on towards climax.

opposite above: Using your mouth on your partner is the best way to say you find them delicious.

opposite centre: Sensual connections continue even after climax.

opposite below: Tantra can help you to delay the finish of lovemaking, again and again.

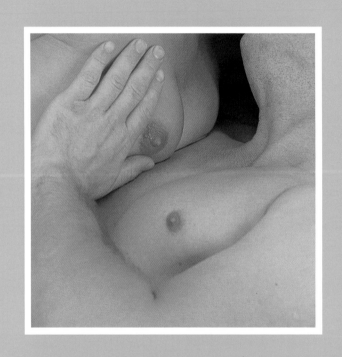

THE TANTRIC RITUAL

4

AT THE HEART OF THE PHILOSOPHY IS THE TANTRIC SEX RITUAL. TANTRISM PUTS SEX AS A CENTRAL ASPECT OF LIFE BY SEEING ENJOYMENT OF SEX AS A CELEBRATION OF LIFE ITSELF AND A WAY OF LINKING TO THE GODS, THE UNIVERSE, AND TO YOUR PARTNER.

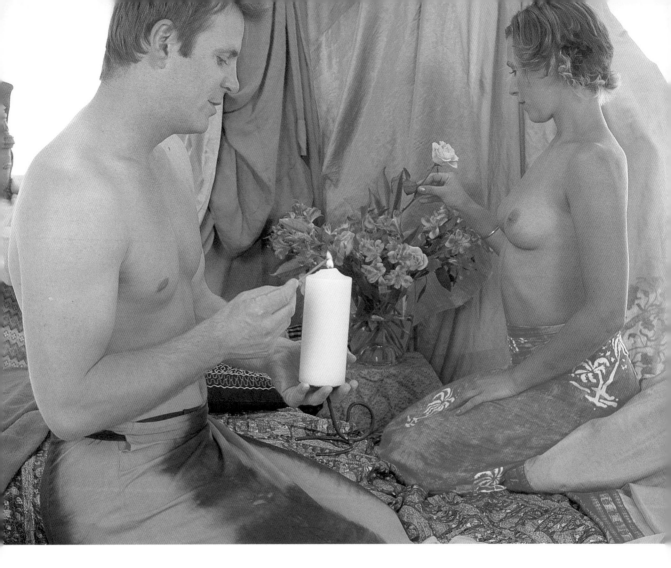

The Tantric Sex Ritual is the way you bring together all aspects of your life. The ritual allows you to take a journey – an extended exploration – through the preparation of the scene to the first steps, the initial touches, and onto a sexual connection that builds up into an explosion of ecstasy and beyond. In the *Kama Sutra*, Vatsyayana describes the day in the life of a citizen who follows the arts of love, and he makes it quite clear that a couple who wish to reach heights of passion need to prepare and take their time in pleasing themselves and each other. He not only details the way an evening of love should proceed, but starts with the moment they get up in the morning.

Vatsyayana sets out how his ideal couple may follow a rite that brings them together in passion. For a start, he suggests that you should be as well versed in as many of the Sixty-four Arts as possible (see also pages 20–23). To win over the man or women of your choice, you need to entertain and delight them. The Tantric arts of love are not about going out for a night on the town, getting drunk and then falling into bed with each other. They are about cherishing and valuing, about recognizing your whole selves and weaving the essence of each other together. They should involve teasing and tantalizing, stretching the moment so that both of you experience maximum pleasure over the maximum period of time. In many ways, in Tantric sex, the journey is more important than the arrival. In Vatsyayana's eyes, communication and self-expression were vital aspects of a fulfilling relationship. The more you knew, the more skills and arts you had at your fingertips, the more interesting a person you became and the more entrancing you would be to a partner. In each sexual encounter you have, all five senses as well as the mind should be engaged, and the Tantric Sex Ritual sets out to do just that. Nowadays, we may wish to alter the list of 'essential skills' in the Sixty-four Arts: for mineralogy, you might substitute knowing how to send e-mails; for chemistry, you might prefer to know how to programme a video recorder or operate a video camera! The point is that you should be interested and interesting, and be prepared to talk and share your knowledge and feelings with your partner.

SETTING THE SCENE

When getting ready for the Tantric Sex Ritual, pace yourself, building up anticipation, expectation and arousal slowly and gradually. Not only will you extend the experience, you will also heighten it, and devotees often report whole-body orgasms that exceed anything they may have experienced before.

Prepare an area where you have time and space to concentrate on each other and to invest in a sense of reverence and expectation. Comfort, warmth and security are all-important when planning your surroundings for Tantric sex. So, too, is choosing a location that immediately informs you that pleasure and physical excess are on the agenda – and are not only allowed, but also encouraged. Set aside a space that will be used solely for you and your partner to engage in the ritual. In an ideal world, a special room would be kept for this, and this alone. Unlike Indian royalty, few of us have mansions or palaces, so choose somewhere that will be private and that can be made special for a period of time. If you have children, you may need to send them to family members or friends for the night or, if they are older, encourage them to go out with their friends and leave you alone for the evening. To create a safe, private, closed environment, lock the doors and close the curtains or shut the blinds (shades). Turn off mobile (cell) phones and take the phone off the hook, or turn on the answer machine and turn off the sound.

Clear a space to spread out, either by removing furniture to another room or by pushing pieces to the edges of the room. A bedroom can be used, but while much of what you do together can take place on a bed, the firm surface of the floor is essential. Bedrooms, including guest bedrooms, are only advised if they are large with a good amount of floor space; otherwise, use your living room. Throw a covering over the television, and the computer if you have one in the room, so you will have no temptation to think about outside influences. You will need to be relaxed and warm, whether wearing light clothes or none at all, so turn up the heating or light a fireplace if you have one.

Sensuality and spirituality

Decorate the room in various textures and colours so it speaks to you of sensuality and spirituality. For the sensual side, gather cushions or pillows and lay them out on soft, comfortable throws, blankets or thick towels. Use warm colours, such as vibrant reds and passionate purples, lively yellows and earthy oranges. For the spiritual side, think of the colours of the chakras – red, orange, yellow, green, sky and indigo blue, and purple – and try to make sure they are all represented somewhere. If you can, hang drapes that are sumptuous and colourful, and if possible, richly woven and decorated; sari material or muslin (cheesecloth) panels are especially effective. The most ordinary and dull room can be transformed with a flame-coloured muslin curtain draped across the window or doorway, billowing in a breeze.

Flowers and fragrance

The sense of smell is particularly important in the ritual. Vatsyayana, for instance, suggests to sprinkle the sheets, cushions or pillows with perfumes and fragrant flowers. You could burn incense or essential oils, spray the room with a room essence or your favourite scent or cologne, and set out bowls of potpourri. Musk, myrrh, frankincense, rose, patchouli, sandelwood and jasmine are said to be particularly sexy scents, but choose according to personal taste. Fresh flowers are vital, not only for their scent but to bring in an air of freshness, of life and of nature, so whatever is in season would be good choices. Roses have romantic associations and can be beautifully scented, as can freesias, lilies, hyacinths and sweet peas. Floating flowerheads in bowls of water will make the association with life and nature even stronger.

Tantrikas often create an altar, upon which they may place a sacred statue or symbol, and lay candles, flowers, oils and incense, to help them in their ritual. Although creating a sacred area is not entirely essential, it can serve as a spot on which to focus and meditate. A coffee table or the floor may also be used as a place for all the things you need and will use.

Candlelight

As well as colour and comfort, warmth and security, and scent and flowers, you need to light your setting. It is important not to be in darkness. Tantric sex does not take place in an atmosphere of shame or secrecy, where people seek to hide themselves or what they are doing. Tantric sex is all out in the open, but you do need atmospheric lighting. For several reasons, candles are an asset. One is

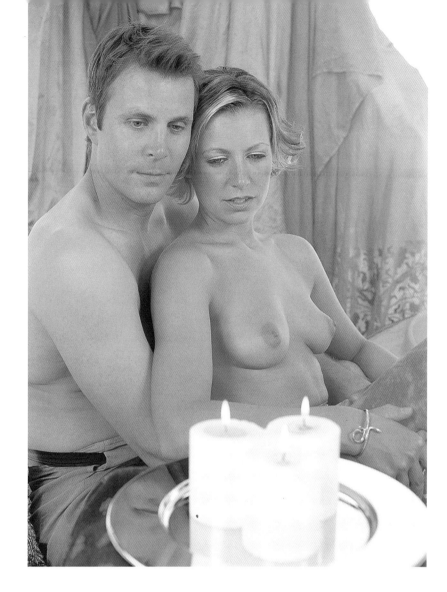

left: Pamper your senses
and light up your sex life.
Candles, altars and flowers
can also create a focal point
for the meditative stage
of the ritual.

because you can use scented candles to stimulate all your senses. Another is that candles add warmth as well as light. A third reason is that candles are a valuable aid to meditation. They flicker and vary, which helps you focus on the meaning of the changing moment. Candlelight gives just the right amount of illumination – enough to see by, but not too much to glare and be off-putting.

Above all, a room lit by candlelight has an interesting effect on the eyes and what you and your partner see when you soul-gaze (see page 74). The pupils of the eyes react to dim light by expanding to allow as much light as possible to be gathered in. By candlelight, the pupils will be dark and wide. This is significant because the same thing happens when you become sexually aroused, and your pupils expand. We are all aware that when we get excited our genitals and nipples react by becoming engorged and enlarged, but not everyone realizes this happens to the eyes as well. Even if you were not familiar with that fact, your body knows it and part of your mind does, too. So when you look into your partner's eyes, you will notice if these are the eyes of someone turned on by you. And nothing has the power to stimulate you more than being faced with apparent proof that your partner is stirred by you. So, dim the lights, throw a scarf over the shade, or switch them off and scatter small nightlights and votive candles everywhere. Candles can be placed in specially bought holders or on everyday saucers, or in preserve jars, bowls or glasses. Set them on tables, bookshelves, windowsills and on the floor. Hang up lanterns or make your own using preserve jars strung with thin wire.

The foods of love

In the *Kama Sutra*, Vatsyayana says that when the citizen receives his woman, he should invite her to take refreshment and drink freely. Spend some time preparing a plate or tray of favourite little nibbles with your partner, such as dips with chips or vegetable sticks, slices of small fruit and other finger foods. Have your favourite drink at hand, such as wine or beer, fruit juice or mineral water. Some foods are reputed to be aphrodisiac – to have the power to arouse you. Pomegranates, for instance, are thought to be the fruit of love, and these 'love apples', not your garden-variety Granny Smiths, are said to have been the fruit that tempted Eve in the Bible. The rich, ruby colour and grainy texture of the pomegranate fruit is thought to resemble the sumptuously coloured flesh of a woman's vagina when she is aroused, and so eating the fruit is meant to be sexually stimulating for women. Oysters, with their salty smell and slippery texture, which also resembles a woman's parts, have long been reputed to arouse men. Bananas and asparagus are also thought to act on men – to have them stand up in imitation of the erect shape. Chocolate, too, is a well-known aphrodisiac. Choose your own favourites and get ready to feed each other.

Accessories and oils

To enhance the atmosphere, select music to play that you both like – slow and smoochy, with a beat or a mixture of styles. Set out items and props to pamper, thrill and pleasure each other, such as massage oils and creams, feathers and sponges, brushes and combs, and wash cloths and towels. You may like to decorate your bathroom, too, by putting candles on every surface and laying out warm towels, fragrant soaps, shampoos, body oils and creams.

Scented bath and massage oils can be purchased, or mix your own custom-blend. For massage oil, mix three parts of an essential oil to every 100 parts of an unscented 'carrier' oil, such as sunflower or almond oil. Essential oils recommended for a sensuous experience include black pepper, cardamom, jasmine, juniper, orange blossom, patchouli, clary sage, rose, sandelwood and ylang-ylang, however some can be dangerous if you are pregnant, so check the label. A few drops of an essential oil can be added to a warm bath, or mix six to ten drops in a tablespoon of vegetable, nut or castor oil before adding to the bath. Make bath salts by combining a few drops of essential oil with 150 g (5 oz) bicarbonate of soda (baking soda) and 75 g (2½ oz) powdered orris root. Store in an airtight jar and add a handful to a warm bath when needed. If you plan to shower, wrap a handful of dried herbs in a square of muslin (cheesecloth) and use to rub over your body or hang from the showerhead. For a stimulating mixture, choose basil, bay leaf, lavender, lemon verbena, lovage, meadowsweet, rosemary, sage or thyme. For a relaxing blend, use catnip, camomile, jasmine, lime flower or vervain. Rose petals are romantic and can be placed in sachets or sprinkled in baths or on bedding.

below: Sharing food prepares you for other pleasures to come and allows you to engage in the intimacy of feeding one another.

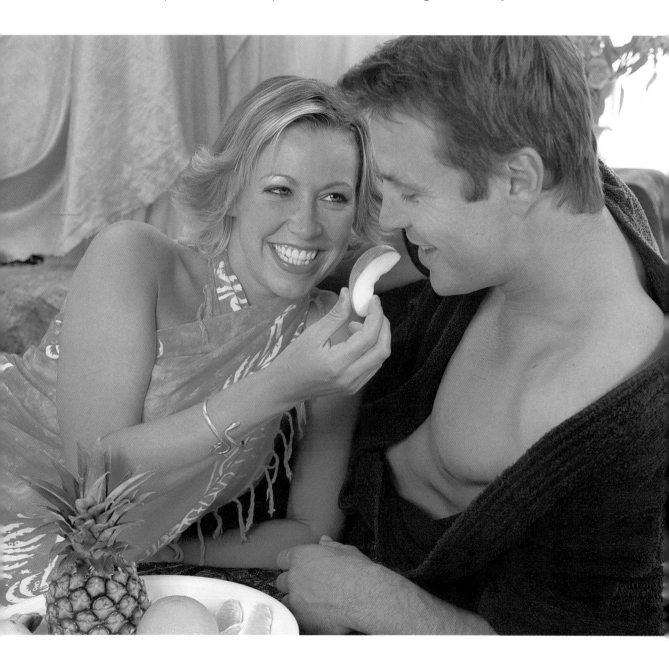

PREPARING YOURSELF

Once you have arranged the room, it is time to prepare yourselves. Part of getting ready is a question of awareness – knowing and acknowledging that you and your partner plan to come together and celebrate love and all it means to you, and to give each other pleasure. From the time you get up that morning

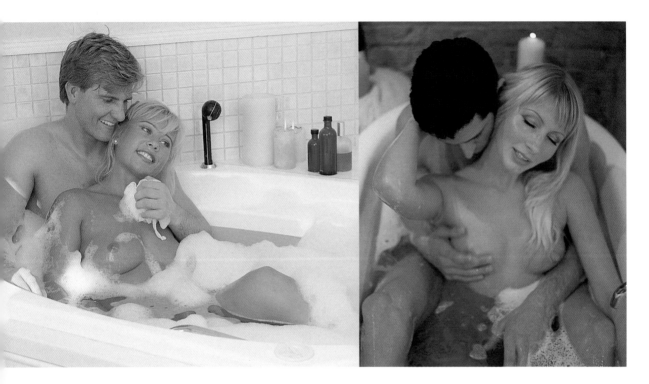

above left: Bathing together is symbolic as well as arousing, allowing you to get in touch with your bodies.

above right: Take a candlelit bath, using soap to cherish and excite each other.

opposite: Pat each other dry, exploring the contrast of rough texture against smooth skin, before applying fragrant oils or creams.

to the moment you both settle down to enjoy the Sex Ritual together, you may be leading up to the moment. Far from spoiling it, this awareness only adds to your readiness and so to your eventual pleasure. Acknowledge in the morning that this is what you plan to do later that day. Remind each other as the day goes on – by kissing and touching each other if you are together, or with phone calls, e-mails or text messages if you are apart.

Bathing and dressing

Preparation as you enter the rite may involve bathing. Washing – separately or together – has two important symbolic functions. You dissolve away the cares and demands of your day and get ready to present your partner with a new, fresh, revitalized you. But you also take the opportunity to cherish and honour yourself. If one of you is at home before the other, you may want to be ready and let your partner catch up. Or choose to start the ritual by bathing together.

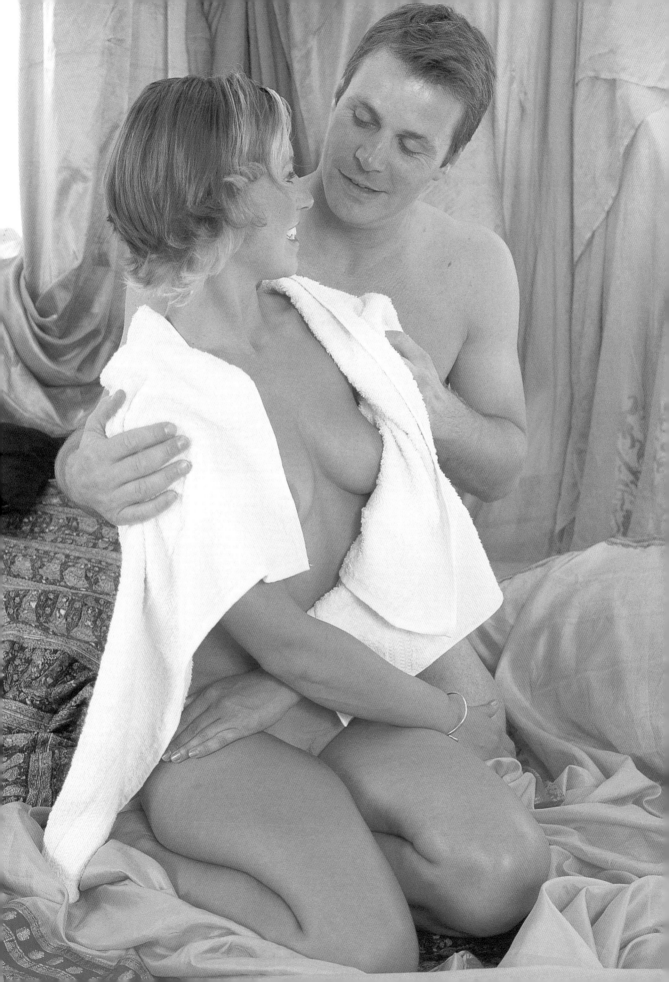

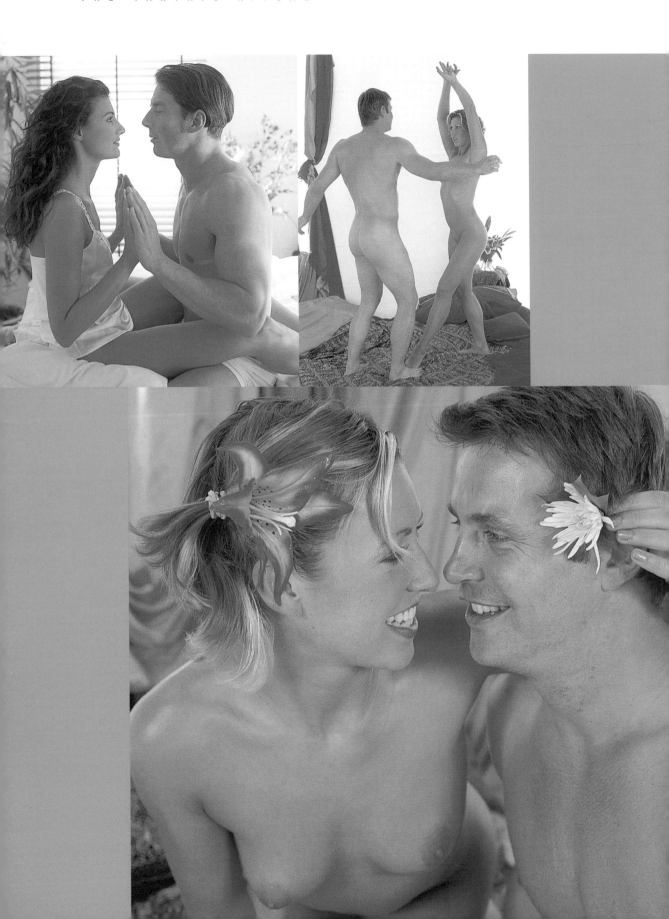

When showering or bathing, make a point of passing your own hands over every part of your body with reverence and love. Appreciate yourself and, in doing so, get ready to let your partner appreciate you, too. Use a razor or cream to make yourself as smooth as you like. Apply a favourite soap or wash, bath oil or gel and take a moment to relax and prepare. Having washed, dry yourself – or dry each other – and then take an aromatic oil or cream and smooth it all over, or let your partner do it for you. Anoint every part of yourself, telling yourself that you and your body deserve special treatment. Spray yourself with a favourite scent, cologne or aftershave and dress in loose, comfortable clothing. If you can, select something that has a sensuous or luxurious feel, like silk, soft cotton or muslin (gauze). A T-shirt and light joggers or boxer shorts, or a slip, chemise or a sarong are comfortable, sensual choices.

above left: Begin with a centre of calm by soul-gazing and limited touching.

above right: Use dance and movement to become in tune with your partner and get the blood flowing.

below: Indulge in the pleasures of scent, texture and adornment.

BEGINNING THE RITUAL

Settle down comfortably to calm and centre yourself before the storm. You can do this together, side by side or face to face. You may like to sit a little apart from one another, to prepare for later, up-close delights. Arrange yourself in the most comfortable position to meditate (see pages 29–30). You may be cross-legged on the floor, kneeling with your legs doubled up underneath you or sitting on a chair. Either close your eyes or fix them on a candle flame or other object that helps you focus. Use a mantra, aloud or in your mind, or play music or nature sounds to help you concentrate. Meditate for 20 minutes or more, and then slowly come to your feet and shake yourself back to awareness. Wait for, or join, your partner. Play music and move your body in dance, at first alone but gradually in time and in tune with your partner so that soon you are dancing together. Dance with your partner until you feel your blood circulating throughout your body and you are in step with each other.

Now is the time to begin to indulge and treat each other. Take the tray of snacks you prepared earlier and offer them to your partner, feeding them their favourite titbits with your fingers. Pour them a drink and present it, lovingly and attentively. Relax on the cushions and pillows as if you were Sultan and Sultana, Prince and Princess. Entertain each other by playing a game, reading to each other from a book or magazine you may want to share or telling each other about something that interested or amused you during your day.

Groom each other, paying attention to your bodies. Let your partner brush your hair, leaning back against them as they cosset you. In return, manicure their nails or give them a gentle foot rub. You may like to ornament your partner's body in some special way. Darken their eyes, colour their lips, or even touch up their nipples with make-up. Apply a temporary tattoo or Mehndi (henna) tattoo somewhere only you will see it, such as the backside, hip or

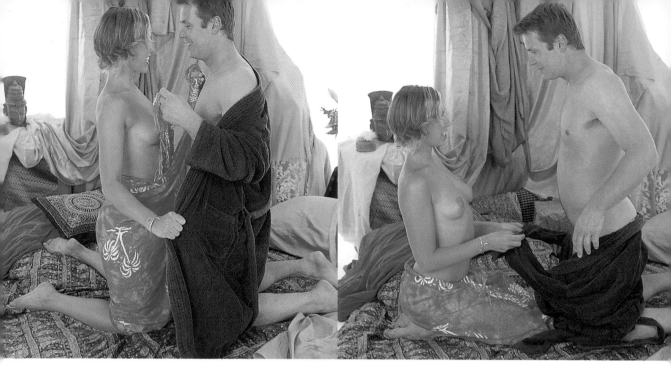

even near or on the genitals, undressing each other slowly as you go. If you like, take some nail scissors and trim their pubic hair into a shape that pleases you both – short and sexy, or by making the top line heart-shaped.

Massage and visualization

When you are both relaxed and revelling in each other's company and attention, warm oil or cream in your hands and, starting at their feet, begin to massage your partner. Gently and carefully remove any remaining clothes so they are naked and massage their whole body, touching every part, doing it with love and sensuality, but without sexual desire at this stage. Honour, respect and adore your partner's body, and when you have massaged them entirely, let them do the same to you.

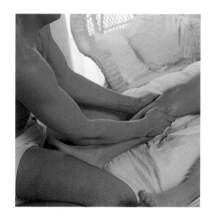

above: Taking the time to massage your partner from head to toe shows that you care for and honour them.

Once every muscle has been kneaded, every bit of skin has been caressed and the blood is singing through your veins, arrange yourselves in a sitting or kneeling position, facing each other. Look deep into each other's eyes and soul-gaze (see page 74). You may find that your sexual desire peaks sharply as you do this and you want to connect. Share a kiss; as many and as deeply as you like. If desired, start to touch each other with sexual intent.

Begin to pass your hands over your partner's body. As you caress and touch, use visualization to increase your sexual arousal. Press your hands together and rub around the chakra points, envisaging the energy vortexes. Picture each gate and its colour (see pages 16–17 and 33–37). Imagine energy being stimulated by the contact between you, moving from each chakra through the nadis to the crown as Kundalini force is awakened and spirals up. Feel the energy that you breathe in through your chakras and pass to each other. Awaken and stimulate that energy through eye-to-eye contact and by

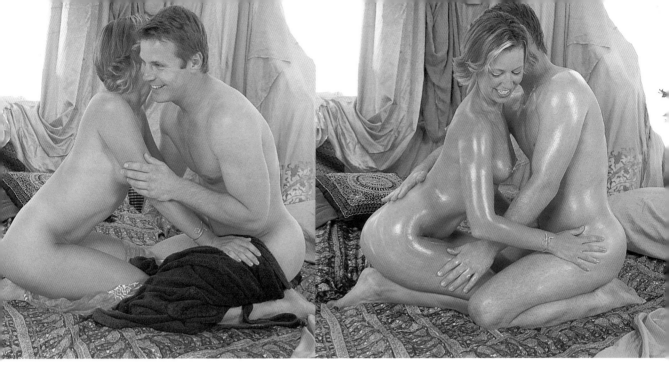

using your hands, fingers and tongue to touch. Then hold each other closely, aligning your chakras and using deep breathing to let energy flow between you. Pay special attention to the rhythm of your partner's breathing. Gradually begin to inhale as they exhale, exhale as they inhale, while visualizing your chakras alternately taking in and breathing out energy, bringing yourselves into synch. Become so attuned to each other's body language that you are an extension of one another, each able to follow at once what the other does.

Remember that you don't have to accept all the Tantric beliefs to make this work for you. One couple may see the ritual as two people getting in touch with the cosmos, embodying in themselves the spirit of Shiva and Shakti, connecting with the dynamic energy in the universe and passing such force between them. Another couple may just view it as a way of paying each other undivided attention and communicating honestly and fully as they get closer and more intimate.

THE LANGUAGE OF TOUCH

Touch your partner, encouraging them to show you what they like, what they want and where they would best appreciate your touches. Instead of feeling that, by guiding you, they are implying you don't know what you're doing, see it as a form of communication; you can't read their mind, and each act of love is a fresh discovery, a new way of doing it. If you don't ask or accept direction, both of you will lose direction. Take your partner's hand and guide them to the places where you would like to be touched at this time, and show them how you want to be touched.

Start with gentle strokes, using the tips or flats of the fingers, the palms or the backs of the hands, and build up. Use your tongue and lips, or pleasure your partner using something soft or scratchy. Feathers or fur gloves, a silk scarf, a bath loofah, sponge or back brush can all be used to stimulate and excite.

far left: Tease and promise by unwrapping each other like a present.

left centre: Tell your partner that you like what you see as you slowly disrobe and reveal each other.

right centre: Touch, caress and discover what pleases both of you most.

far right: Use fragrant oils or creams to anoint and adore.

top left: Let the energy flow between you through deep breathing and meditation.

top right: Build up from gentle stroking and kissing to using your teeth and fingers to arouse and excite.

below: Set yourself the goal of touching every part of your partner's body.

Pain and pleasure

If you like, and only if you both agree, explore the boundary between what hurts and what delights. In the *Kama Sutra*, Vatsyayana describes in detail the ways lovers can bite and scratch, the better to arouse and excite each other. He recommends using teeth to nip, leaving 'the line of points' when small portions of the skin are marked, or 'the line of jewels' when all the teeth are used, leaving an extended imprint. And he says, you can leave marks with nails in the armpit, on the throat, breasts, lips, torso or thighs, in the shape of a circle, a half moon, a line or 'a peacock's foot' or 'the leaf of the blue lotus'.

Vatsyayana also describes ways of 'striking with passion', recognizing that some couples find spanking a stimulating part of lovemaking. You can use the tips of your fingers, the palms of your hand or a loosely curled fist – but gently. Certainly, scratching, nipping and smacking can be intensely exciting, but you and your lover will need to find out and agree between yourselves how far to go and whether you want to do it hard enough to leave marks. This part of sex is not about violence and abuse, which would be anathema to Tantric principles, but concerns how much consenting adults decide to take pleasure to the boundaries of pain. You always need to check what pleases the other and only go as far as the person taking the spank or nip really wants to go.

Taking your time

Remember, the keys to Tantric sex are respect and sharing, and taking your time. In most ordinary sexual encounters, the race appears to be on when couples begin to touch each other in a sexual way. Both may find themselves drawn, irresistibly, to each other's genitals; men home in on their partner's breasts and between their legs, and women touch their partner's groin. And before they know it, it's all over. So part of the Tantric Sex Ritual is to pace yourself and set yourself the goal of touching *every* part of your lover's body, not simply the obvious, sexual areas (see also Games to Play, page 94). The interesting result is that you will find that nongenital areas respond dramatically, and that prolonged lovemaking can sensitize all areas of the body. Tantrikas say they can orgasm simply by soul-gazing, by aligning chakras, or by stroking an ankle, a knee or an elbow. But in fact, you don't want to reach the peak of sexual arousal at this early moment in the ritual. What you do want to do is to allow both of you time to feel loved, appreciated and worshipped.

When you feel yourself getting turned on enough to climax, take a break. Sit back and caress each other with love and affection, but without passion, and offer each other something to drink or to eat to relax you. It may take some practise to learn how close you can get to the point of no return, but you can do it. Tantrikas suggest you can continue turning up the tension, increasing desire but holding it at bay, for literally hours at a time.

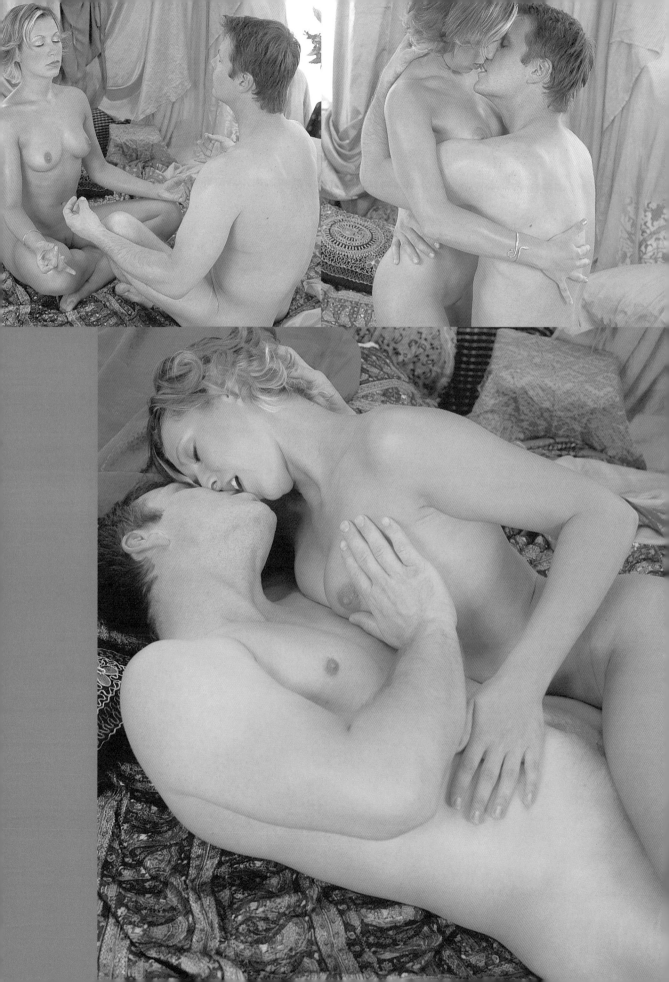

Games to Play

Stroke, caress, lick and arouse every inch of each other's bodies, and employ props and game-playing. Drip wine or hot chocolate onto your bodies and lick it away; stroke cream or honey onto the skin and suck it off. Play kissing games by passing a bit of fruit back and forth between the lips, or ring the changes of hot and cold by trailing an ice cube down your partner's chest and stomach, then mopping it up with a cloth wrung out in hot water. Put a bottle of massage oil in hot water, just enough to warm it, and then trickle the sensual liquid in an erotic stream over your partner's body, paying special attention to nipples and genitals. Alternate touching erogenous areas with stroking and brushing the feet, hands, back, stomach, arms and legs.

BEING WITHIN

At some point (and you may find yourself flowing into it without actually realizing the moment), you and your partner may wish to move on to introducing his lingam into her yoni. You may call this 'penetration', seeing it as the man entering and taking the woman, or you may refer to it as 'engulfment', viewing it as the woman enfolding and taking him inside her. The difference may simply be whether you choose to have Shiva or Shakti in command at first, and these roles are entirely flexible throughout the course of your time together.

Tantric sexual positions, as explored in the next chapter (see pages 98–111), do more than simply add spice and interest to lovemaking. Each position has a significance and a reason. As a result, experimenting with different poses – the man on top, the woman on top, both lying on their sides or standing – is both enlightening and stimulating. Again, the whole point is to take your time and enjoy the journey as much as, if not more than, the arrival at any destination. Instead of picking one position and staying with it, flow from one to another, seeing what each gives to you and does for the two of you together. This gives you opportunity to experiment with new positions and fresh pleasures, which will make your sex life and relationship more satisfying in the long run. Concentrate each moment on the moment, and on each other and the pleasure you are giving and gaining from your lovemaking.

RIDING THE WAVE

Tantrikas talk in terms of 'riding the wave'. As you approach orgasm, it feels like a wave of pleasure that picks you up, carries you on and deposits you, breathless and spent, on the beach of post-climactic bliss. Fast and furious sex can be satisfying, but it can also be a bit premature. One of you – and it is usually the woman – may be left behind as your partner races ahead in a climax that comes quickly and disappears just as instantly.

When a couple learns to 'ride the wave', various results can happen. Orgasm can be controlled and delayed, which means that both of you get the chance to have your pleasure while making love. Riding the wave also means that desire and sensation can build up over an extended period of time, so that when the orgasm does come, it is that much more dramatic and breathtaking. It may also mean that both of you can surf on the crest of passion and response, dipping in and out of that 'point of no return', letting the sexual tension mount and mount. The more times you repeat the build-up towards climax but turn back at the last moment, the longer you will both last and, when it comes, the more mind-blowing the climax will be. The key to riding the wave is to take

below left: Various positions have different significance and results. Allow yourself to flow from one into another.

below centre: Crest the wave of passion to let go in complete pleasure.

below right: Controlling and delaying orgasm may mean she comes many times.

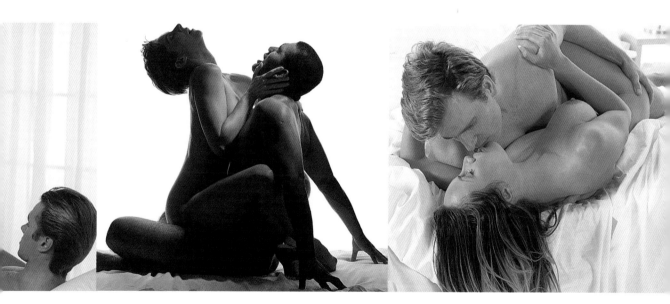

a break whenever you feel yourself reach the threshold of orgasm. Stop what you are doing, focus on your breathing and visualize your sexual energy being drawn inwards as you reach for calmness and serenity.

As your ritual develops, you may wish to reach a point where she climaxes, but he still holds back. Most woman are capable of achieving several, if not many, orgasms and still continue to enjoy sex. As you become skilled in the arts

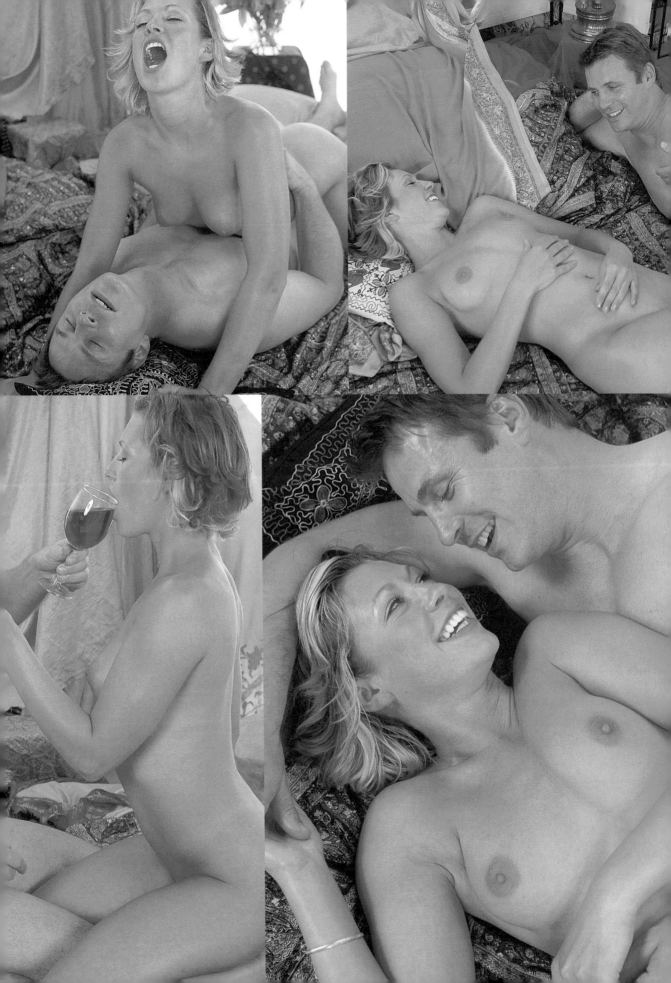

of Tantric sex, you may reach a stage where both of you become multi-orgasmic, and are able to share several orgasms before the man is unable to go on. Of course, even when he does come, lovemaking can last. Both of you may choose to continue caressing and touching, and using tongues and lips to please each other. Tantric sex encourages women to let go in sex and orgasm, to enjoy being abandoned and passionate, to seize the moment and grasp pleasure with both hands. Vatsyayana recommends a whole litany of sounds lovers may utter to show passion and enthusiasm. You don't need to learn his sounds – let loose and find your own!

RELAX AND CHILL OUT

Once both of you have orgasmed, lie close together and enjoy the intimacy. You may want to kiss, talk and laugh about what you have just shared, and to tell your partner what parts were especially good for you. You can lie face to face, and chakra to chakra, or cuddle up spoon-fashion. Relax by playing some soothing music and listening to it together, feeding each other from your goodies tray again or sharing a glass of a favourite drink. You may find that one orgasm is simply the prelude to another, and you can ride the wave onwards for some time.

Eventually, you will come to a point when you have had enough of the peaks of pleasure and are now ready to sample more relaxed and less energetic ways of showing and sharing your love. In the *Kama Sutra*, Vatsyayana suggests that the couple returns to the bathroom to cleanse themselves and anoint each other with creams and oils once more. This may be a signal for the two of you to lie back in each other's arms, and to relax and chill out. Satisfied, in tune and energized by your experience, you may want to spend some time enjoying the afterglow before settling down to sleep, curled up together, or easing into another activity.

top left: Screams of pleasure and delight can urge him on.

top right: One orgasm can be a prelude to more, but take a pause if you want to delay.

bottom left: Share a glass of a favourite drink and enjoy being in the moment.

bottom right: Lie close and share your special, intimate relationship.

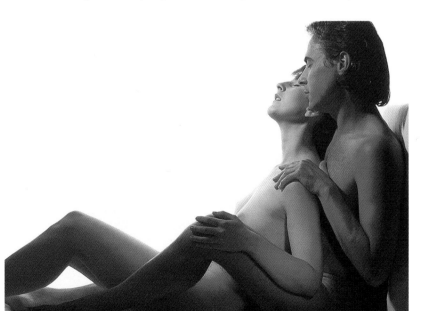

left: Spend some time enjoying the afterglow of satisfied love.

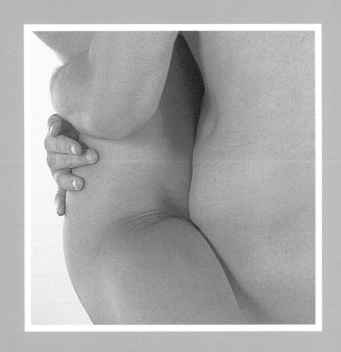

TANTRIC SEX POSITIONS

5

ONE OF THE MOST IMPORTANT ASPECTS OF TANTRIC SEX IS THE DIFFERENT POSITIONS TANTRIKAS TAKE WHEN MAKING LOVE. AS FAR AS MOST OF US ARE CONCERNED, A VARIETY OF MOVES ADD SPICE AND INTEREST TO YOUR SEX LIFE.

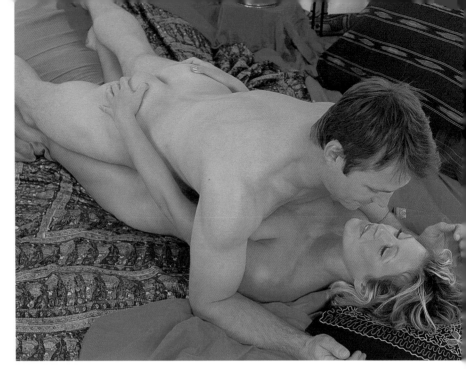

right: Face to face in the
Clasping Position, the man
is in control and in charge.

Some sexual positions are better for fast and furious sex, whereas others are
more suited to slow and long union; some allow men to enjoy themselves to
the full, and others encourage women to find their pleasure. However, in Tantric
sex, sexual positions have a larger role: they are believed to help move energy
around the body. The positions aid the partners to embody the male principle,
'purusha', and the female principle, 'prakriti', and to achieve identification with
the god and goddess, Shiva and Shakti, who are the manifestation of these
principles – Shiva being the male and Shakti the female.

The positions of the lovers' bodies during sex are believed to be magical
and mystical, enabling the couple to transmit energy, and enliven and revitalize
themselves and each other. The ritual positions of lovemaking are known as
'mudras'. Just as dances have intricate and exact forms, with preordained hand,
feet and body positions, so do the mudras. As well as energy, the different
lovemaking positions encourage the flow of body fluids, which are believed to
be sacred, and which the man seeks to conserve in himself and encourage in
his partner (see page 19). In some sexual positions, the male principle is
uppermost, allowing him to be dominant, while in other mudras, the woman
is active and powerful and in control. In yet other positions, both partners share
their energy, which flows between them.

Vatsyayana, in the *Kama Sutra*, describes a variety of lovemaking positions,
including the Clasping Position, the Pressing Position, the Splitting of a Bamboo
and the Congress of an Elephant. The most popular, and certainly one of the
most powerful, Tantric positions for sex is when the couple face each other. Face
to face, you can kiss while making love, which is a profoundly intimate contact.
You can also gaze into each other's eyes, communicating your wishes and
needs, and sharing understanding and emotions. Within the basic heading
of face-to-face positions, there is a wide range of different ways to have sex.

FACE TO FACE: MAN ON TOP

The most common sexual position is with the man on top. This position, known to most of us as the Missionary Position, allows the man to have freedom of movement and to experience the sense of mastery and strength that comes with the male being in the ascendant, dominant position. To balance this, he should remain sensitive to his partner's needs, using his arms to support his weight and making sure she receives as much pleasure as he does. This position gives them both advantages: the man is able to reach the woman's breasts and clitoris, even if he can use only one hand to caress her.

In the masculine dominant pose, you can use the Clasping Position, where the man lies on top of his partner with his legs on top of hers, both having their legs stretched out straight. He can support himself on his elbows and she can hold his buttocks or press down on the small of his back to steady and control the timing of his thrusts for her pleasure. A variation of this, when both partners stretch their legs out in a 'Y' position, can also be exciting.

below left: Lying side by side, he has freedom of movement to caress her.

below right: Pressed between her legs, she can pull him in deep and close.

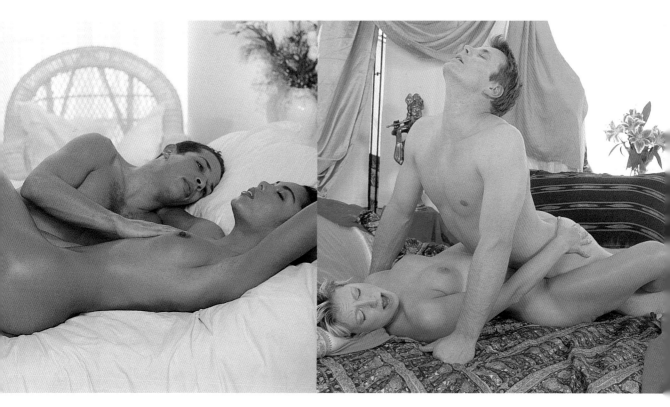

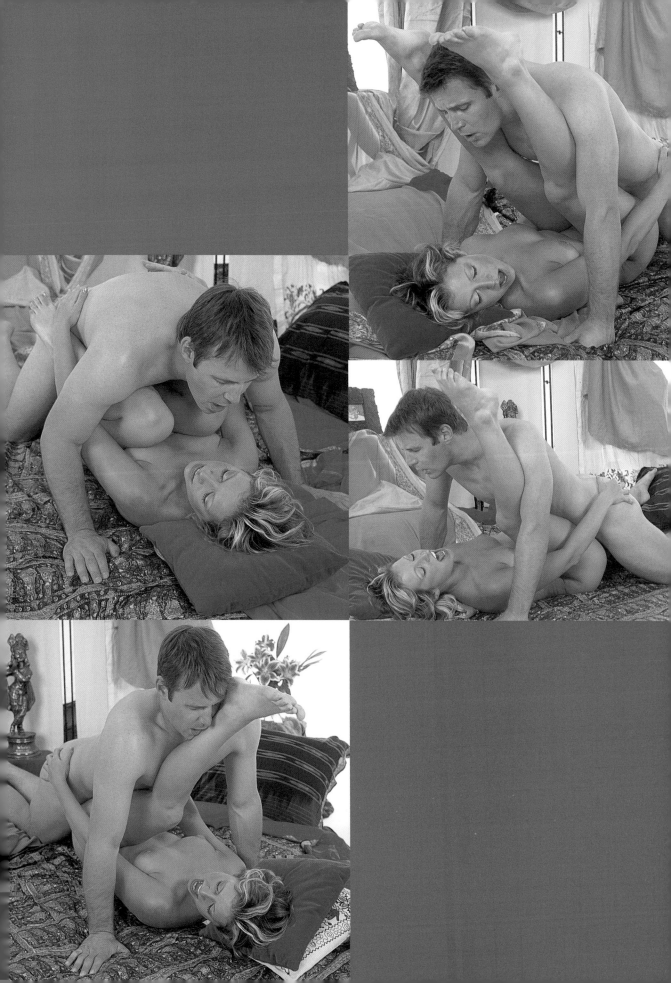

Pressing Position and the Mare's Position

The Pressing Position is one type of man-on-top positions. In this, the woman grips her partner between both her thighs, curling her feet and ankles over his calves and holding him firmly. The position allows the woman to have some control over her partner's movements, so she can make sure his thrusts coincide to her timing and the angle of his entry is satisfying to her.

While lying together in this way, women can also practise contracting and holding the muscles around their yoni, or vagina. Gripping his lingam with her yoni is said, by Vatsyayana in the *Kama Sutra*, to be learned only with practise, and is sensationally exciting for the man. He calls this the Mare's Position and it is also effective for the woman, as it allows her to contract and flex the muscles and tissue around the vagina, transmitting sensation to the clitoris and so bringing her to orgasm. To learn how to do this, imagine trying to hold back a stream of urine, letting it stop and start, and practise repeatedly (see also pelvic tilt exercises, page 116). Keeping his lingam gripped inside her yoni is said to best allow him the opportunity to benefit from her amrita and sexual energy.

Variations

Another exciting variant of the man-on-top positions is when the woman raises her legs and wraps them around her partner's waist, or raises them even further, resting her shins and knees against his chest, which Vatsyayana calls the Pressed Position. The position opens the woman up to the man, offering ease of penetration. The Yawning Position, where the man is on top and the woman has her legs raised and her ankles resting on his shoulders, takes this one step further and is particularly good for deep penetration.

In the *Kama Sutra*, Vatsyayana recommends a position called the Splitting of a Bamboo. In this, the man supports himself on his hands while his partner lifts one leg over his shoulder, the other one stretched out. She then changes legs, stretching the raised leg out and raising the stretched one to the shoulder, and continues to alternate one leg and then the other. The most difficult of the face-to-face, man-on-top positions is the one Vatsyayana calls Fixing a Nail, which he says you need to practise. The man supports himself over his partner, while she has one leg raised and resting on his head.

However, in the early days of experimenting with sexual positions, it is worthwhile looking at variations that satisfactorily stimulate the woman's clitoris. One useful type of man-on-top position that helps achieve this is to place a cushion or pillow under her hips, lifting her up so that he can alter the angle of entry to find a position that suits her as well as him. Vatsyayana recommends the Widely Open Position, where the man balances on his knees as well as his hands, and the woman raises her hips off the surface, lifting both of them up and in doing so, pressing her clitoris against his body.

top right: The Yawning Position allows the man to have maximum penetration.

left centre: The comfortable Pressed Position leaves her wide open to him.

right centre: Splitting the Bamboo, where the woman alternates her raised legs, adds variety and interest.

left bottom: Fixing a Nail needs a little practise, unless you are flexible and adept at more difficult contortions.

Churning

The only problem with the Missionary Position is that, while it is intensely pleasurable for him, it is also quite a strain. The man needs to make sure he doesn't press down too heavily on her breasts and ribcage, and this means he must hold himself up on his arms. As this is tiring, it may hurry him along to

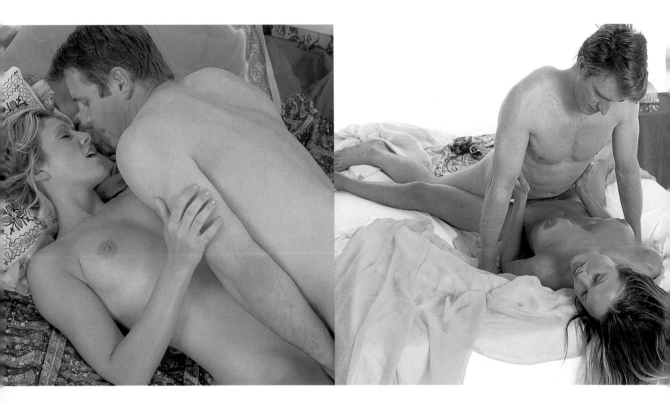

above left: Churning is pleasurable for both partners and can hit the G-spot.

above right: Legs in the 'Y' position add variety to the classic man-on-top position.

his orgasm sooner than either of them would wish. Many women say that they do not orgasm from lovemaking in this position on its own. The strength of Tantric sex is that, by involving so many other aspects of lovemaking, women do find that even man-on-top positions become satisfying.

One variation that helps women reach ecstasy in the more conventional man-on-top positions is described by Vatsyayana as 'churning'. In this exercise, the man holds and guides his penis as he penetrates, and then thrusts inside, his partner. He directs his penis not only inside her vagina, but also so that it strokes and rubs up against the upper side of her yoni, an area known as the G-spot (see also page 123). The G-spot corresponds to the same spot that is the prostate in the man. Although some women have no special sensations when this area is touched, others find it intensely sensitive and report that when it is stimulated, they experience not only strong orgasms but ejaculations, and fluid pulses out of the vagina as they come.

FACE TO FACE: SIDE BY SIDE

Face to face, but lying on your sides, allows long, slow sex and the sharing of sexual energy. The easiest position is the one Vatsyayana called the Twining Position, in which the couple lie side by side with the woman's upper thigh thrown over the man's body. You can also lie thigh to thigh, holding each other's hips to remain in close contact with each other. In another variation, the man may bend and bring his knees up towards his chest and his partner can lie inside his legs, her weight on his lower leg.

FACE TO FACE: UPRIGHT POSITIONS

One important element in Tantric sex, emphasized in the *Kama Sutra*, is that sex doesn't only – if at all – take place in bed with the lights out. Indeed, participants are encouraged to have sex in a special place that may have a couch or bed, but isn't necessarily the place in which they sleep. It also follows that sex isn't something you *must* do lying down. If the aim of Tantric sex is to encourage Kundalini force to awaken from the base of the spine and ascend to the Sahasrara chakra, it follows that making love upright helps the journey.

below: For long, slow sex, get into the side-by-side Twining Position.

An upright position that may be enjoyable for both partners is when the man kneels upright between her legs, or even stands. By lifting her pelvis with his hands or by placing a pillow or cushion underneath her hips, he can alter the angle of entry to find a position that suits them both. For example, the man can kneel upright between his partner's legs as she lies back, with legs wrapped around his waist. But better still may be when she lies back, raising and resting her feet up against his chest. His hands are then totally free to caress her breasts and clitoris, or to stroke her feet while he kisses and sucks her toes.

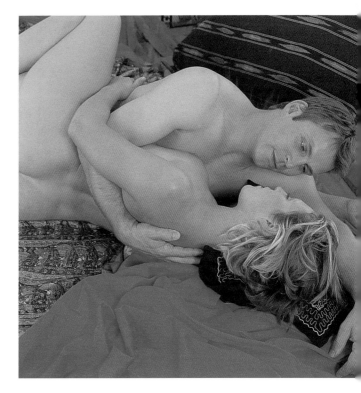

Couples can make love sitting facing each other, he with his legs stretched out and she with her legs wrapped around his waist as she sits in his lap. In this position, they can hold each other closely so chakras align and touch. Or, they can lean back, caressing each other's bodies while soul-gazing. He can cross his legs with one or two feet up on his own thighs in the Lotus Position (see pages 40–41) as she sits close in his lap with her legs around his waist.

Suspended and Supported Congress

Another variation of face-to-face positions is with both partners standing up. If you are the same height, you can stand genitals to genitals, but if one partner is smaller and lighter than the other, they can wrap their legs around the heavier and taller partner's thighs while being held up themselves by their bottom or thighs. Needless to say, this is quite a tiring way of making love that needs plenty of practise to manage successfully. Vatsyayana called this position Suspended Congress, while he named sex standing up and leaning against a wall or some other support, Supported Congress.

FACE TO FACE: WOMAN ON TOP

The woman is considered to be the active force in Tantric sex. In Tantric belief, Shakti (the female) moves, while Shiva (the male) is acted upon. Squatting astride and in the lap of the man, knees raised, mimics the position often shown in representations of the deities making sacred love, and women on top puts the female principal in the ascendant. The advantages become clear: with the woman lying on her partner, the man has his hands free to stroke her body, caress her breasts and nipples, and to gently touch her clitoris. By taking away the need to support himself, the position also allows him to save his strength and, in doing so, last longer. But the main advantage is that, by having control of the speed, strength and angle of movement, the woman can discover the point at which the clitoris is best stimulated by body-to-body contact. Women find that if they ride quite high on their partner, they are able to give themselves sensations that are particularly strong and satisfying. With the man lying on his back and the woman sitting with his erect penis in her vagina, she can also move in such a way as to bring the penis into contact with her G-spot, which may lead to multiple orgasms.

There are a wide variety of woman-on-top positions: lying full length on top of the man, thighs inside or outside his; with knees raised and feet flat on the floor; with his lingam in her yoni, leaning backwards with her feet underneath his shoulders and her weight supported by her arms. The position can also be done sitting down, with her legs around his waist or thighs. Whether he is sitting or lying, this is a position that gives the man staying power and the woman the majority of control, considerably improving both their pleasure.

Pair of Tongs

With the woman on top of the man while making love, she can hold him in the Pair of Tongs. She does this by gripping and contracting her vaginal muscles, holding him firmly inside herself. In this position, if he can delay his own orgasm while she enjoys hers, according to Tantric belief, he will be imbibing her essence and storing up considerable sexual energy for himself.

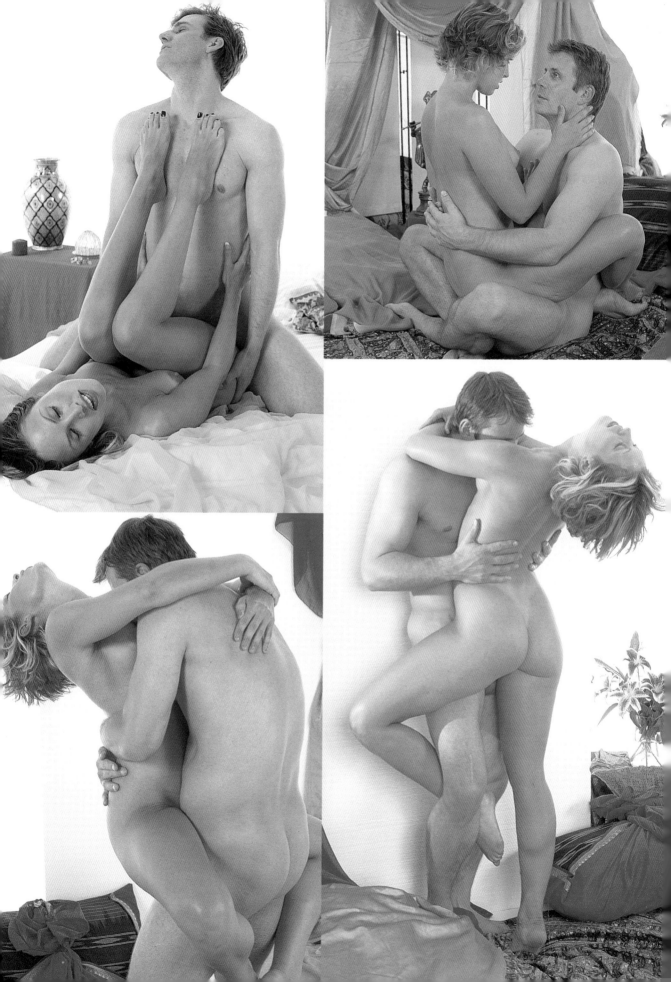

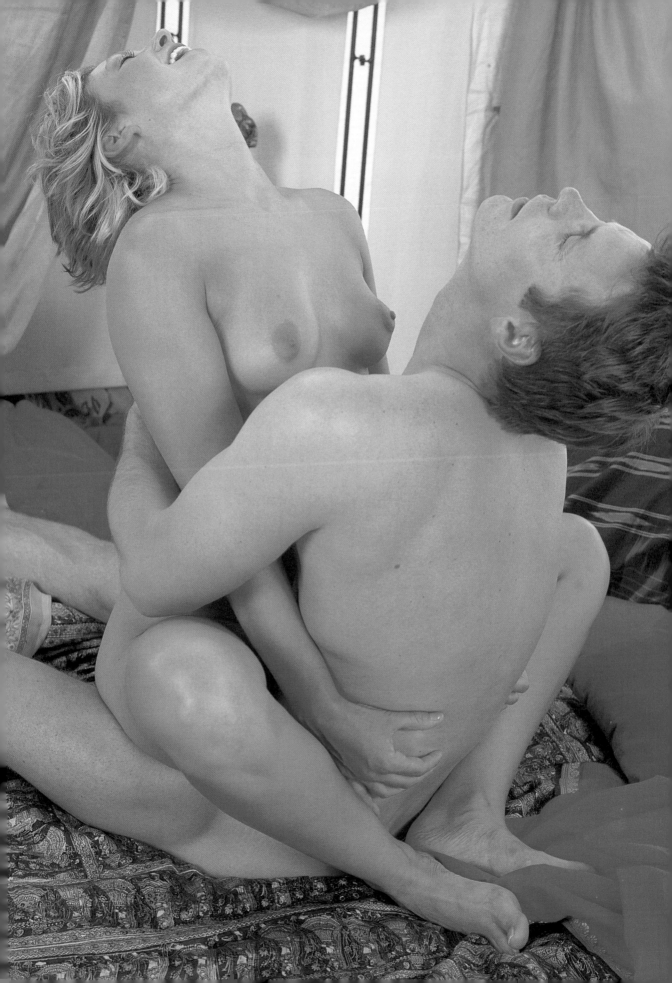

MOUTH CONGRESS

In the *Kama Sutra*, Vatsyayana devotes a whole section to Auparishtaka, or Mouth Congress. Ask men what single sexual variation they would like to add to their lovemaking, and most would vote for oral sex. Although it is this sex act that suffers most from fears and apprehensions, it often gives the most satisfaction. Oral sex can be the greatest compliment you can pay your partner, showing them that you think they are good enough to eat. Yet so many people fear their partners will find their private parts too unpleasant to smell, taste or look at to want to perform this intimacy. In fact, most men or women are turned on by the sight, taste and smell of their partner's genitals, and would be only too pleased to be allowed to show how delicious they think their lover is.

opposite: The female principal in the ascendant, she holds her man in the Pair of Tongs.

below: Mouth Congress says you are good enough to eat.

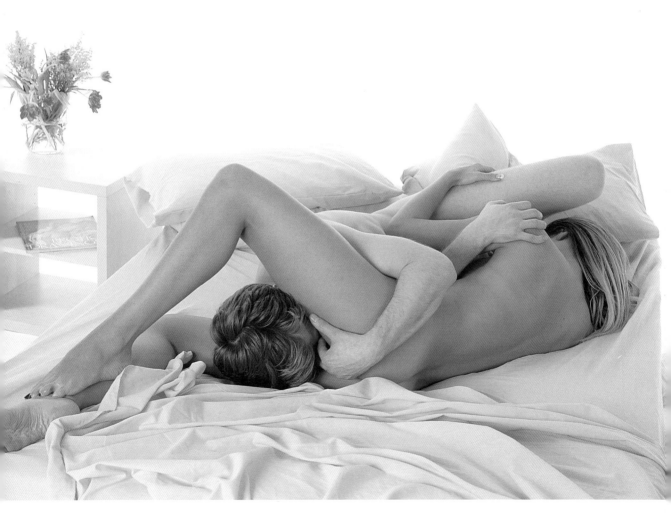

You can kiss, lick and suck – in the *Kama Sutra*, known as 'sucking the mango fruit' – or nibble around your partner's genitals. Some people prefer gentle movements, with their partner using lips and tongue to nudge them to arousal. Start by gently running your tongue around your partner's genitals to see how they react. You may then go on to firmer attention, tonguing and nibbling, or even gently nipping them. Some people enjoy having the clitoris or glans sucked; others like their partner to gently blow on skin that has been dampened by licking. But, in spite of the fact that oral sex is also known as 'blow jobs', you should not blow into a penis or vagina. It won't be pleasurable and may cause a potentially fatal embolism or a nasty infection. You can give each other oral pleasure turn by turn – him on her is known as cunnilingus and her on him is called fellatio. Doing it together, at the same time, is known as '69' or 'soixante-neuf'. Vatsyayana calls the 69 position the Congress of a Crow.

COMING FROM BEHIND

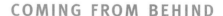

You don't have to be eye-to-eye to make love. Indeed, our early ancestors started off having sex in the same way as much of the animal kingdom, with the male entering from behind, and this is a very practical position. Rear entry makes it particularly easy for both partners to reach and caress the woman's clitoris and bring her to a full orgasm. Full, deep penetration can be achieved in this position and, by moving her legs to various angles, the woman can enjoy a range of different sensations. Many women find rear-entry sex is the best position for stimulating the G-spot (see page 104). With the woman lying on her stomach or bending over, legs apart and hips rotated slightly upwards, she can move her pelvis to make contact with the G-spot.

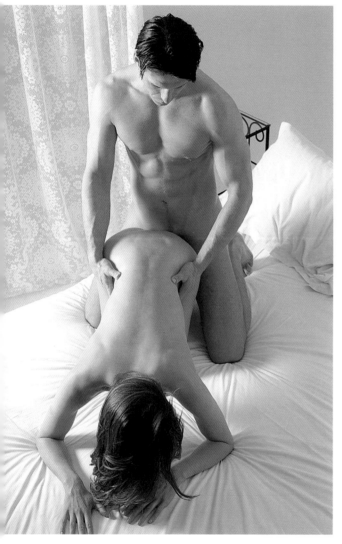

above: The animalistic rear-entry positions give sex an extra kick.

Variations

You can come from behind in all sorts of ways, from standing up to lying down. A favourite position is one in which the woman lies face-down with her upper body propped up over pillows or cushions and her backside raised. The man kneels between her legs and enters her. He can also stand behind her as she leans over the side of a bed or chair, and he can also hold her legs up as he stands between them. She can sit either on his lap with her back fully to him, or turned halfway round, with one arm around his neck. Finally, you can have rear-entry sex lying side by side, spoon-fashion. The man may lie on his side with his thighs curled up and under her backside, with the woman lying against him and both legs flung over his.

Rear entry, or as we call it in the West 'doggy style', may be felt to be wicked and animalistic, giving it an extra kick. Vatsyayana described ten different rear-entry sexual variations, each named for an animal you would imitate. From the Mounting of an Ass, through the Congress of a Cat and the Rubbing of a Boar to the Jump of a Tiger, you can have fun and visualize yourself becoming one with the animal kingdom and the cosmos by being each animal as you make love. Rear-entry sex can be done lying down, sitting up or standing, and can also be enjoyable in a bath or shower. Indeed, the *Kama Sutra* lists several animal-named sexual positions that can only be carried out in water, such as the Congress of an Elephant (see right). You can splash about to your heart's content, using soaps and oils to make the experience even more sensuous and exciting.

ETERNAL CHANGES

There are literally hundreds of possible variations (some say 521, to be precise) in which to make love. You can ring eternal changes by shifting your bodies, bending or straightening legs, sitting up, leaning over, or supporting yourself on elbows, arms or knees. A difference can be made by using pillows, chairs or walls to prop you up or drape yourself across. Some sexual positions give you a thrill because of your attitude towards them – they seem rather naughty and, therefore, more exciting. However, others actually afford increased sexual sensation to men, women or both. Tantric sex encourages you and your partner to explore as many positions as you like as you both proceed through the Sex Ritual. Each position helps you achieve bliss by enabling you to awaken Kundalini force, or by helping the two of you discover what arouses and satisfies you best. In the dance of love, the more steps you practise, the better you become at entrancing, arousing and delighting yourself and your partner.

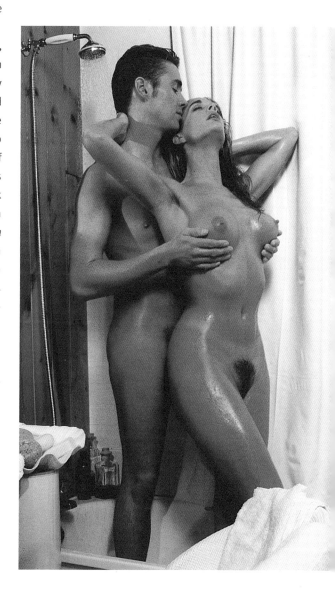

above: Some positions, such as the Congress of an Elephant seen here, need water.

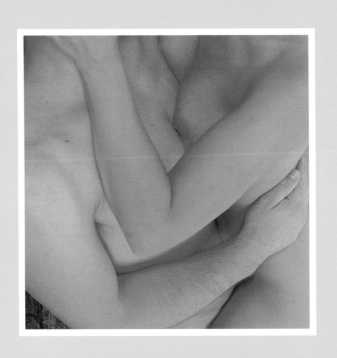

SEXUAL ECSTASY

6

ORGASM – THE 'BIG O' – TENDS TO BE THE GOAL OF MOST SEXUAL ADVICE BOOKS AND SCHEMES. WE WORRY ABOUT WHETHER WE ARE ABLE TO ACHIEVE OR GIVE OUR PARTNER GOOD ORGASMS. ONE OF THE DIFFERENCES THAT CHARACTERIZES TANTRIC SEX AND SETS IT APART FROM OTHER EROTIC SYSTEMS IS THAT ORGASM IS NOT SEEN AS THE BE-ALL AND END-ALL OF LOVEMAKING.

The Tantric approach to orgasm has two important advantages. One is that it encourages, helps and allows you to enjoy the journey as much as the arrival. All too often in lovemaking, couples charge ahead into penetrative sex, cheating themselves and each other of full enjoyment. At best, you each have an orgasm but one that arrives quickly and abruptly. At worst, his climax is hurried and soon over, while she is left frustrated and unfulfilled. The main disadvantage is that, because you are concentrating on the ending of the encounter (the climax), you miss out on the delights you could be relishing as you progress. Goal-oriented lovers often forget to caress and touch. They pass on too quickly to have time to suck and lick, stroke and admire, cherish and pamper all the other parts of the body, except the ones that seem to contribute to the Big Bang. It isn't simply that the whole thing is over so soon, it's also that you leave whole areas of each other's body unstimulated, untouched, unaroused. Couples who indulge in slow and extended sex soon find that the pleasure derived from stretching out the experience may be even better than the sudden and soon-over sensations of an instant climax. Slowly, teasingly and gradually massaging your partner from the toes to the crown of the head can arouse sensations that may be even more ecstatic than if you went straight for their genitals and brought them to orgasm. The second advantage of the Tantric approach is that when orgasm does come, it is likely to be far more widespread, more sensational, more explosive and far more satisfying than an orgasm achieved through two minutes of foreplay and one minute of intercourse.

Tantric sex helps develop your sexual skills. Following the Tantric Sex Ritual allows you to pace your lovemaking and use your imagination. Knowing there is a set of rules to abide by, a recommended form to fit into, allows you to rein in previous headlong and uncontrolled behaviour and make it a special and lengthy occasion. But as well as simply extending the moment, Tantric sex can help you learn skills and abilities which really add to the lovemaking experience. Tantric sex can help you to learn how to control your orgasms, how to have whole-body and extended orgasms, and help you enjoy multiple orgasms.

CONTROLLING YOUR ORGASM

For many couples, orgasmic control is about ensuring that she comes before he does. In Tantric sex, orgasmic control focuses on both partners delaying their final satisfaction in order to extend and expand their delight. We all go through a fixed set of reactions when becoming sexually aroused to orgasm, which is called the Sexual Response Cycle (see page 69). It is fixed in that you usually proceed from the arousal phase, through plateau, to orgasm and into resolution. But what is variable is that, if interrupted, you may not have an orgasm. When orgasm does not occur and you stop lovemaking or masturbating at that point, resolution takes longer. When that happens, tissue such as the genitals and nipples, which are engorged with blood, may take half an hour to relax and return to their usual size and shape, leaving you feeling sore and frustrated.

Another variable is that you can have enormous influence on the length of time of the arousal phase, and over what happens after you come. The famous sex researchers, Masters and Johnson, said that the arousal or excitement phase can last from several minutes up to hours; plateau phase can last from 30 seconds to 3 minutes; orgasm from 3 to 15 seconds; and resolution from 10 to 15 minutes. They also pointed out that, after orgasm, men experience a refractory period, during which they cannot be stimulated to further orgasm and that this can last from several minutes to many hours. The refractory period, they found, does not occur in women, who, in fact, may be able to have 20 to 30 orgasms during one session – barring simple exhaustion! The researchers also confirmed that the younger the man, the shorter the refractory period. However, men may also notice that in times of heightened excitement, such as the first sexual encounter with a new partner or love-making with an established partner in special circumstances, the refractory period may diminish. The man may then find he can make love up to several times in one night, enjoying many repeated erections and recurring orgasms. The basic trick is to harness the circumstances that make this happen, and have them under your complete control. The better the lovemaking is overall, the more intense the experience, and the more likelihood there will be a shorter refractory period.

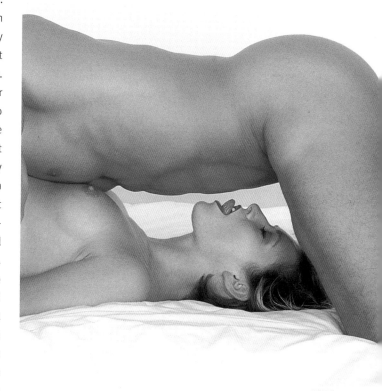

Women often learn not to delay their orgasms, because of anxiety that if they put it off, they may miss out altogether. If your partner is likely to come quickly and then roll over and go to sleep, this may make sense. But, on the other hand, if you and your partner are joining forces to expand your loving practice, and coming together to enhance both of your lovemaking skills, it need not be a fear. Even if, in the early days, he does climax before both of you are ready, sensual stimulation with the mouth, tongue and lips, hands, fingers, palms and toes can continue until the woman is satiated and satisfied. Try the following strategies to delay your climax until you both decide that it is the right time to come.

above: Use the mouth, lips and everything else to give sustained pleasure.

Pelvic tilt exercises

Both partners will find that pelvic tilt exercises can help you control and enjoy orgasms. Lie down on a firm surface with your hands resting comfortably at your sides, knees bent and feet flat on the floor. Tense the stomach muscles so they are firm and make sure your lower back is in contact with the floor. Focus your mind on your pelvic region, specifically the muscles surrounding the woman's vagina and the prostate in the man. The best way of doing this is to imagine

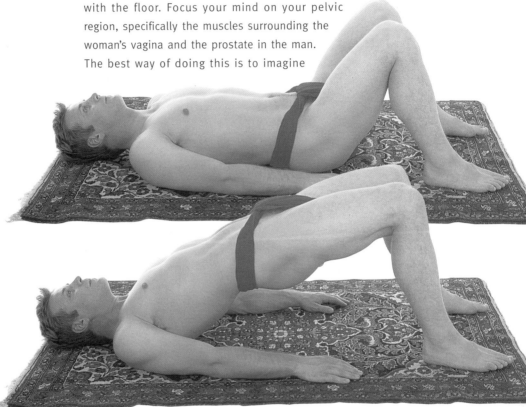

you want to pass water, and then take action to stop it. The muscles around the vagina or around the prostate will tighten. Now inhale and lift your hips off the ground. Count to ten as you hold the muscles tight, but continue breathing in and out, and lower yourself down on an exhalation. Repeat ten times, and perform the exercise regularly to tone up the pelvic muscles.

Toned pelvic muscles contribute to your general health as well as enhance sexual performance. Women are less likely to suffer prolapse of the womb if their pelvic muscles are strong and both sexes are less likely to suffer incontinence, a common problem with child-bearing and aging. Sexually, both partners may discover their ability to enjoy climax is enhanced. Flexing the pelvic muscles can help a woman to become aroused and to have an orgasm (see the Mare's Position, page 103); a man may find it enables him to keep his erection and hold off ejaculation for longer.

KNOWING YOUR TRIGGER POINTS

It is not enough to be aware that stroking his penis or stimulating her clitoris, or the nipples or other sensitive areas, may lead to sexual arousal and, finally, to orgasm. You need to know what leads to your arousal and orgasm. Everyone is different, and loving couples should explore and experiment to discover exactly what it is that turns their partner on. But you need to know your own body and its particular responses, too. Take the opportunity to settle down and examine yourself intimately (women will need to use a hand mirror to do this). Look at your genitals and learn how they look and feel. Dispel any negative feelings you may have that your genitals are too big or too small, too hairy or sparse, too smooth or too wrinkled. They are yours alone and are perfect in their own way.

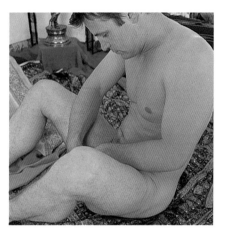

Now begin to stroke and manipulate your body, finding what pleases and excites you. You can do this in bed or in the bath, using cream or oil to make the sensation even more pleasant. Don't confine your touches to your genitals, but watch to see how they change and react. Men will find the penis lifts and enlarges as the scrotal sac tightens and the balls tighten up against the body. Women will see the inner and outer lips change colour, shape and size, the vagina become moist and the clitoris may be visibly larger. If the woman puts a finger in her vagina, she may feel the vagina lengthen and flare out inside, at the top. Both sexes may find their nipples and the darker area around them enlarge and stand out. As the plateau phase starts, both will see their skin flush and women will see their breasts enlarge. The colour of the vaginal lips will deepen, moisture from the vagina will increase and breasts will swell in size. During orgasm, she may feel her vagina

above and below: Both partners need to know their own bodies and trigger points in order to give and receive pleasure and excitement.

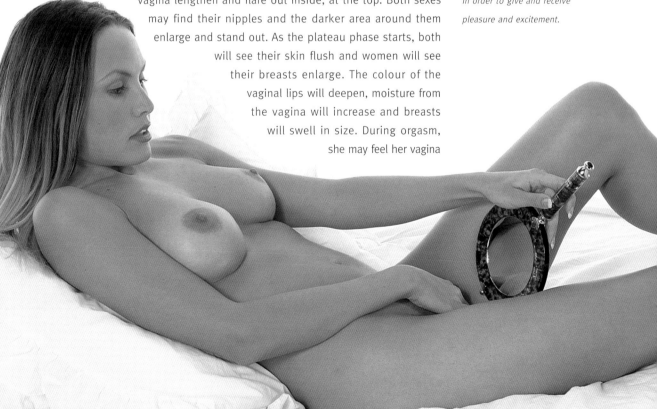

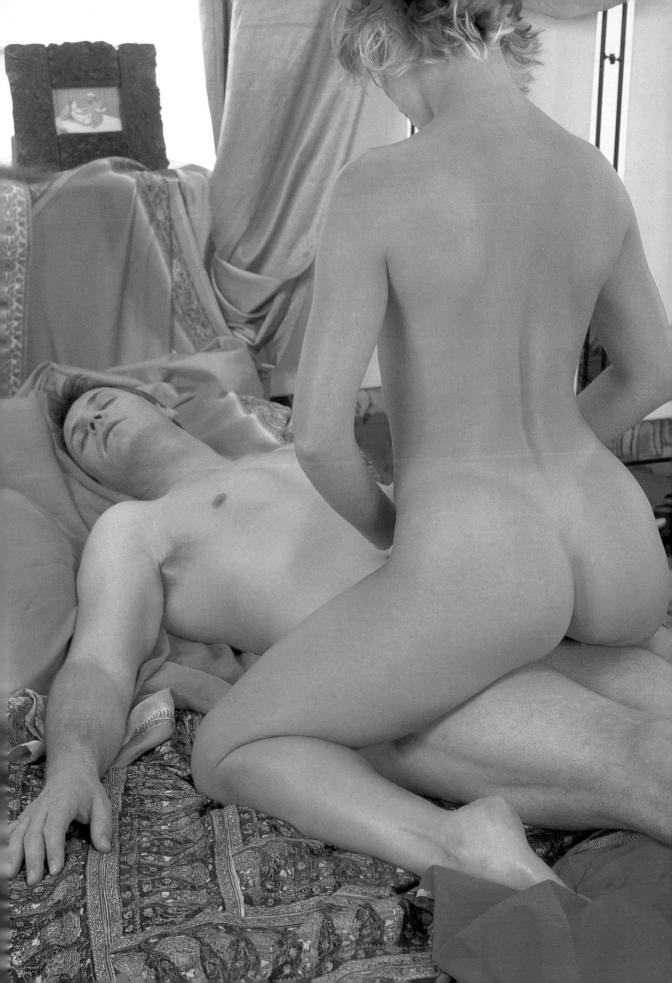

and back passage clenching and her womb contracting. He will feel his back passage contract and pulse as he ejaculates. During the 10 to 15 minutes after having sex, both will be able to see their skin return to its usual colour, as everything that has enlarged or deepened in colour returns to normal.

Once you know the signs, you can monitor yourself during sex. If you have seen and felt what happens when you get excited, you can learn what touches, caresses or forms of stimulation bring it on. Being aware of what happens when you reach the plateau stage – the 30 seconds to 3 minutes before orgasm – allows you to pull back when you see or feel it advancing or beginning.

KNOWING WHEN TO STOP

Both men and women can feel the moment just before climax takes over and becomes out of control. In men this is known as the point of ejaculatory inevitability. What happens is that the prostate gland and seminal vesicles, areas that produce semen and sperm, contract, forcing seminal fluid along the tubes to the penis and out. The man can feel when this is about to happen, but once underway, he can't stop it. Women, too, can feel changes, as the vaginal lips flush a deeper colour and the uterus and vagina start to flex and contract. If you concentrate as you experiment with self-pleasing, you can learn when these sensations are about to begin as you are making love to your partner.

If you and your partner are making love and want to delay orgasm, slow down and stop as soon as you detect the early trigger signs. Tell your partner that you need to slow down for a moment. Rest and wait, and allow yourself to retreat from the point of no return. Stop moving and lie still but close to each other, and breathe together, inhaling and exhaling slowly and deeply. Pick up the rhythm of meditative breathing (see pages 30–32) and concentrate on the sound of your own breath or that of your partner. The technique may sound cold and clinical at first, but once you have tried it out a few times, doing it becomes second nature. Instead of feeling as if this is a halt to the fun, it will become a welcome rest and a promise of pleasures to come.

During pauses, talk with your partner, share the moment and stay close. You may want to offer each other a drink or a slice of fruit, or a warm towel or a cold wash cloth to freshen up. Make this a positive and creative pause in the banquet of delights you are enjoying. The man may well soften or lose his erection, but don't worry, it will come back. Of course, as you and your partner begin to become practised in the art of Tantric sex, the aim will be to let the woman come as many times as she wants, while the man waits and delays. Pauses may allow her to catch her breath after an orgasm and will also help him put off the moment of orgasm. The man may wish to continue giving her pleasure, using his hands or mouth, while letting himself 'go off the boil'.

opposite: Learn to slow down and stop to delay the moment of orgasm and achieve lasting pleasure.

STOPPING EJACULATION

Tantric sex encourages men to learn how to withhold ejaculation altogether. What many men do not realize is that ejaculation and orgasm do not necessarily go together: you can 'come' without emission. If the man doesn't ejaculate, he can often retain his erection and continue having sex. And, if you have an orgasm without emission, you can go on to enjoy another one in the same way, and on through several climaxes until you finally ejaculate. In fact, in many Eastern cultures, it was considered best for both the man and the woman if he only came once every four, or as few as once every ten, times he made love. The advantages are that the man can enjoy extended lovemaking and several orgasms and doesn't have to worry about his partner missing out.

So, how do men learn to separate orgasm from ejaculation? If you look at the four stages of the Sexual Response Cycle – arousal, plateau, orgasm and resolution – you can see that the key is to learn to control the first two phases so you can enjoy part of the third (orgasm without ejaculation) and put off having to go through the fourth phase. Developing better ejaculatory control involves learning two skills. One is the ability to become aware of your own sexual responses, and the other is the ability to do something about it – to make changes in your behaviour so you can take advantage of that knowledge. If you think this sounds too difficult, or even impossible, don't forget that this is what you might have thought as a youngster when told you'd learn how to stop wetting yourself. As a toddler, you learned to become aware of your body's signals that told you when you were about to pass water. You learned to take action, to ask to go to the bathroom. But later on, you also learned how to clench muscles to hold back until you were ready. Ejaculation is the same: first, you learn when and how it arrives; then you learn how to delay it; and finally, you learn how to stop it until you choose to ejaculate. You may not be able to explain exactly what you are doing to manage the delaying process, but practise may enable you to do so. If, at first, you find yourself coming too soon, don't worry. This isn't a failure in your ability to control, but a valuable lesson in what happens to your body.

Delaying tactics

Practising delaying tactics can be done on your own or with your partner, or you can begin by yourself and later have your partner with you. Not only will you learn your trigger points, and pass them onto your partner, but you will become entirely familiar with the changes in your body that precede climax. Take time and set yourself the goal of lasting 15 minutes without coming. Focus your mind on your penis and your pelvic area. With a dry hand, slowly stroke and caress your penis and scrotum. When you feel your arousal level climbing, slow down,

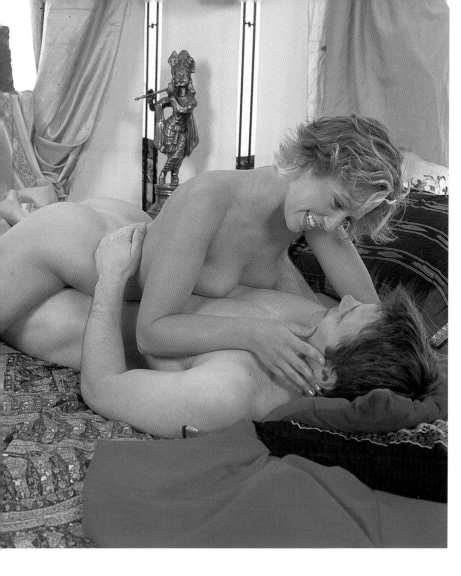

left: Once you can take control, lovemaking can last as long as you desire.

take some deep breaths and stop. Once you feel calm again, continue stroking. Make it last at least 15 minutes before allowing yourself full satisfaction. If you come earlier, simply try for a slightly longer period the next time.

When you are comfortable with the technique and can last for at least 15 minutes every time you do it, begin practising again, but this time slather your hand in cream or oil. You may find that you need to use a lot more control to last! Again, continue the exercise until you can last at least 15 minutes every time you do it. Finally, practise the exercise again, but this time with your partner doing the stroking, and continue until you can hold out every time. You may find that you can control your body's impulses, and without even knowing how you do it, start to have orgasms without ejaculations. If not, apply pressure to a spot between your legs, on the perineum, as you approach the point of no return. The perineum is the smooth area of skin that stretches from behind the penis and scrotum to the back passage. If a man or his partner presses gently but firmly halfway along, just as the man reaches the point of ejaculatory inevitability, it is possible to stop ejaculation but continue with climax. He will experience orgasm, but continue to be erect afterwards and able to move on to new heights.

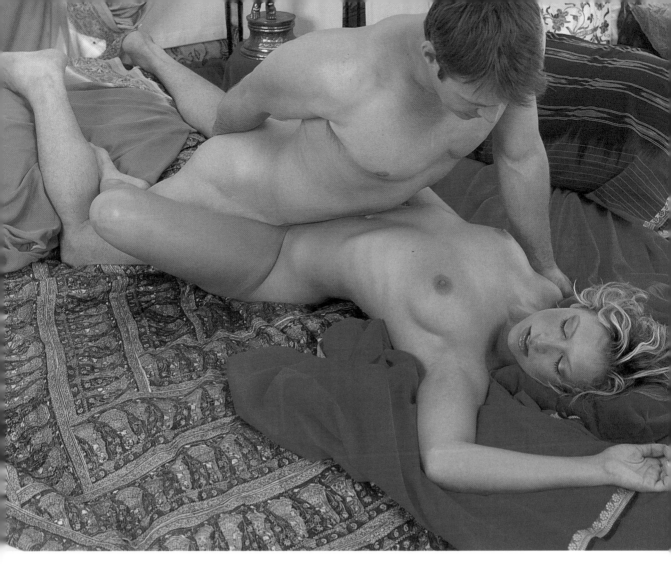

TYPES OF ORGASM

You may think that an orgasm is an orgasm – one is the same as any other. In fact, some climaxes are far more sensational than others. Taking the time necessary, and paying yourself and your partner enhanced attention, will give you the chance to explore a variety of orgasms, from earth-shattering whole-body peaks to the crests and troughs of multiple orgasms.

Whole-body and extended orgasms

Many people say a whole-body orgasm is the ultimate sexual experience. Some describe this as feeling stimulation sweep from your toes to your head and down to your genitals – an explosive sensation that covers every inch of your body. The more you sensitize your body, the more likely this is to happen. Bring your own and your partner's body awake, stroking and caressing, tickling and rubbing, and breathe deeply. Visualizing every part of yourselves coming alive may lead you to feeling every inch of your body responding in ecstasy.

G-spot orgasms

Tantrikas have always known about the area we now call the G-spot, which they consider to be the 'sacred spot'. The G-spot is named after German obstetrician and gynaecologist Ernst Grafenberg, who wrote about it in 1944. He reported on an area in the vagina which, when stimulated, appeared to trigger not only powerful orgasms but also a flow of liquid which was neither urine nor vaginal fluid and which could only be described as female ejaculate. Of course, Tantrikas had always known that stimulating the sacred spot caused the fall of amrita, the female essence. To find the sacred spot, gently insert a finger into the vagina and press the upper wall, about 5 cm (2 in) inside. You may feel a tiny pea- or coin-sized area. Some women find it is most effective when pressed, while others prefer to have it rubbed, and each couple will need to explore for themselves. This can be done with a finger, or the man may find that he can stimulate the G-spot with his lingam by Churning – holding his penis as he enters her and guiding it so it rubs and brushes up against the spot (see also page 104).

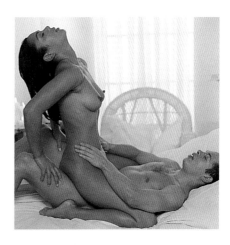

below: Each couple needs to explore for themselves how far they want to go before relinquishing into orgasm.

Multiple orgasms

Because women do not have the refractory period, as men do, they are entirely capable of enjoying multiple orgasms, sometimes in rapid succession. Indeed, women having more than one and as many orgasms as they want and can manage is what Tantric sex is all about. In Tantric terms, the man increases his strength and energy if he delays orgasm while his partner has hers. As she comes, he gains from the effusion of her female essence, whether released in her amrita (ejaculate) or from energy streaming out of her chakras. The more that the man remains in intimate contact, holding her lovingly, sensuously and closely, the greater benefit he may feel. Each successive climax on her part only goes on to increase his force. But Tantric sex may also aid a man in learning the skills needed to help him become multi-orgasmic, too. As well as sensitizing himself to the pitch where his refractory period shortens, men can achieve multiple orgasms if they learn to separate orgasm from ejaculation.

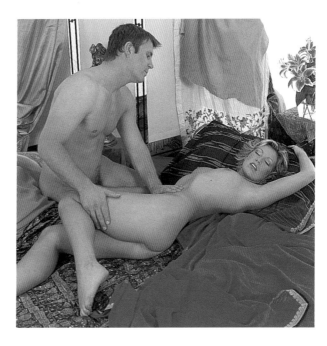

below: Women can have multiple orgasms and some men master the trick, too.

HOURS OF PLEASURE

opposite: Riding the wave
brings extended pleasure
that can last for hours.

When a couple perfects the skills of delaying climax, extending orgasm and enjoying whole-body sensations, they will find that lovemaking takes on a new dimension. Instead of a steady but rapid build-up ending in a burst of sensation, they can learn to 'ride the wave'. This is when they feel surges of excitement sweeping over them, building higher and higher, and going on to new heights instead of dissipating. Each new climax becomes the foundation

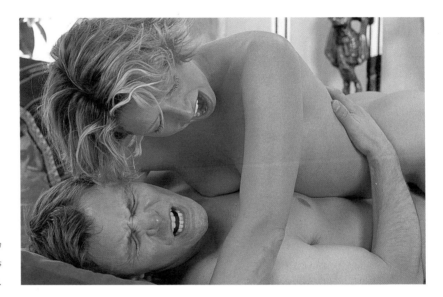

right: Focusing on your own
and your partner's needs is
the ultimate bliss of Tantra.

for yet another. They reach a level where the ongoing and lasting experience is as satisfying and enjoyable as the single orgasm that lasts only a moment and which they may previously have accepted as the best they can expect. Experienced Tantrikas can ride the wave for hours of pleasure that invigorate and delight both partners. Once the pleasure has peaked and died down, those with the skills of love and sex can transfer the experiences they enjoy while making love into their day-to-day dealings. Tantra not only leaves you sexually satisfied, but also with a strengthened relationship, raised self confidence and self esteem. It really is life-enhancing in so many ways.

You do not have to believe in all the tenets and spiritualism of Tantrism to benefit from its key messages – that sex is a core part of life should be cause for celebration and it is a force for good. From following the strategies used in Tantric sex, we can all gain a new way of looking at life and love, and learn skills that enhance our love and sex lives. By focusing, slowing down and concentrating on our own and our partner's needs, we can achieve a lot of the bliss that goes with following the Tantra and create a better partnership.

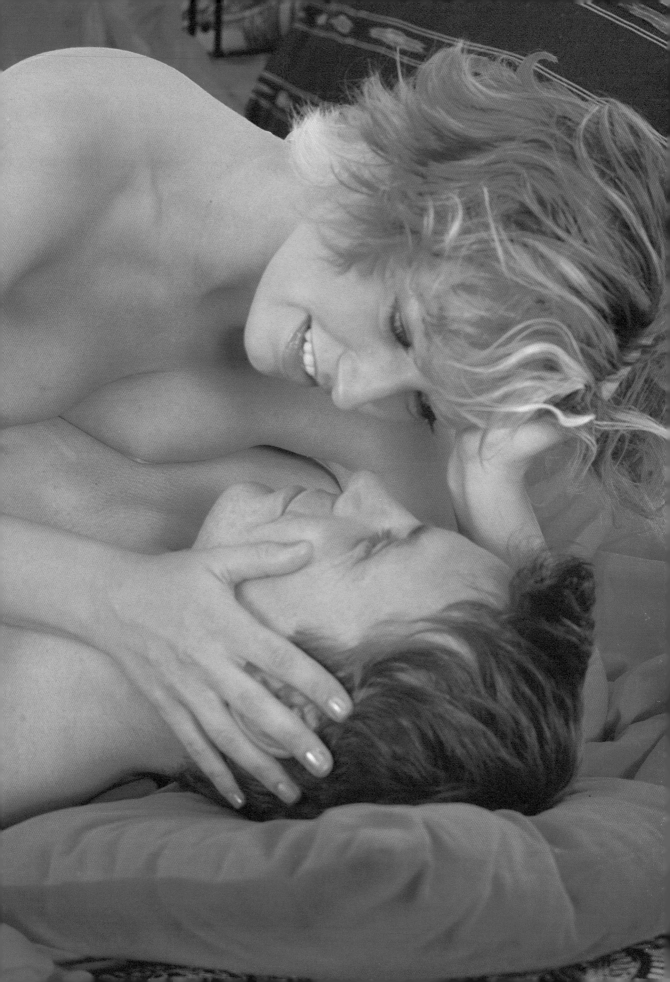

INDEX

affirmation 55
Ajna (Sixth Gate) chakra 17,
    37, 39
altars 82, *83*
amrita (ejaculate) 19, 123
Anahata (Fourth Gate) chakra
    17, 37, 39, 62
aphrodisiacs 84
arousal (excitement) stage
    69, 70, 71, 74, 114,
    115, 120
artha (wealth) 15
asparagus 84
Austen, Jane 20

back, small of 58, 74
bananas 84
bath salts 84–5
bathing 86, *86*, 89, 111
bathroom 84, 97
bedroom 81
beginning the ritual 89–91
    massage and visualization
        90–91
bindu 17, 19
bliss 16, 24, 33, 124, *124*
blood pressure 69
breasts 69, 74, 92, 101, 104,
    105, 106, 117
breath of life *36*
breathing 28–31, 39, 69,
    95, 119
    deep breathing 32, 91,
        92, 121
brushes 84, 91
Buddhism/Buddhists 14, 24

candles *23*, 30, 33, 50, *80*,
    82–4, *83*, *86*, 89
caressing 74, *91*, 97
Cat Stretch, The 44, *44*
chakra asana *7*
chakras (energy centres) 8,
    16–17, *16*, 20, 33, *33*, 36,
    49, 90, 123
    aligning 19, 23, *24*, 39,
        91, 92, 105
    colours 82
    visualizing 33, *33*, 37, 39
    and yantras 41
chanting 23
cheesecloth 82
cherishing women 18, *18*
chilling out 97
Chinese Tao 14
chocolate 84, 94
churning 104, *104*, 123
circle of energy 62, *62*,
    64
Clasping Position 100,
    100, 101
clitoris 57, 59, *66*, 68, 69,
    72, 74, 101, 103, 105,
    106, 110, 117
clothing 89

Cobra, The 42, *42*
colours 82
combs 84
Coming from Behind 110
    variations 110–11
commitment 9
communication 11, 54, 65–6,
    65, 69, 81, 91, 100
concentration 30
Congress of a Cat 111
Congress of a Crow 110
Congress of an Elephant
    100, 111, *111*
Corpse Pose 45
cosmic cycles 24
cosmos 15, 16, 24, 33, 91
creams 50, 59, 84, *86*, 89,
    90, *91*, 97
cunnilingus 110
curtains 82
cushions 82, 89, 103, 110

dance 20, *20*, 23, 46, *46*,
    89, *89*
deep breathing 32, 91, *92*,
    121
Devi *18*
dharma (virtue; religious
    merit) 15
drapes 82

earlobes 57
ejaculation 19, 20, 23, 116,
    119, 123
    premature 55
    stopping 120–21
elbows 57, 74, 92
energy 15, 17
    circle of 62, *62*
    exchanges of 19
    female 18, 23
    male 18
    moving 33, 36, 49
    positive 24
    sexual 8, 18, 19, 20,
        74, 95, 106
    yang 20
    yin 20
erection 69, 119, 120, 121
essential oils 82, 84
excitement stage *see* arousal
    stage
exploring each other 60
    sexual touching 60,
        62–4
eyes 83

facecloths 59, 84, 119
feathers 59, 60, 74, 75, 84,
    91
feet 64, *65*
fellatio 110
female ejaculation 19
female principle (prakriti)
    100, *109*
fingers 57, 74
first principles 54–5
Fixing a Nail 103, *103*
flowers 60, *80*, *83*
flushing 69

focus 30, 31, *34*, 39, 49, 82,
    83, 89, 124
focused exploration 57–9
food/drink 20, *20*, 23, 60, 84,
    85, 89, 92, 97, *97*, 119
foot rub 89
foreplay 49
fur 59, 77, 91

G-spot 19, 104, *104*, 106, 110
    orgasms 123
games 20, *20*, 23, 89, 94
genitals, engorged 115
Grafenberg, Ernst 123
grooming 89

hair brushing 89
half-lotus position 30, 33,
    36, *41*
harmony 13
Harrelson, Woody 6
health 13
heart rate 69
Hinduism/Hindus 14, 24

ice cubes 94
imagination 33, *33*
incense 32, 60, 82
individuality 66

Johnson, Virginia Eshelman
    20, 77, 115
Jump of a Tiger 111
Jung, Carl 17

kama (sex; love) 8, 16
Kama Sutra (Vatsyayana) 8,
    15–16, 18, 20, 80, 84, 92,
    97, 100, 103, 105, 109,
    110, 111
Khajuraho Temple, India *14*
kissing 10, *11*, *71*, 72, 86, 90,
    92, 94
knees 57, 92
knowing when to stop 119
Kundalini energy (life force,
    sexual energy) 8, 16–17, *16*,
    23, 41, *41*, 90, 105, 111

labia 57, 63, 69
lingam 8, 23, 32, 33, 64, 72,
    94, 103, 106, 123
    see also penis
lips 57, *71*, 77, 91, 97
living rooms 81–2
loofah 60, 91
'Look Ma, no Hands!' sex 77
Lord of the Dance 46, *46*
lotion 77
lotus position 30, 33, 36,
    41, 105

male climax 66, 68
male principle (purusha) 100
manicure 89
Manipura (Third Gate) chakra
    17, 37, 39
mantras 23–4, 28, 32–3,
    41, 89
Mare's Position 103

massage 17, 28, 49, 58, 62,
    63, 65, *65*, 90, *90*
    giving a massage 50, *50*
massage oil 84
Masters, William Howell 20,
    77, 115
masturbation 55
    see also self-pleasuring
meditation 16, *16*, 23,
    28–33, *35*, 41, 82, 83,
    83, 89, *92*
Mehndi tattoo 89–90
meridians 62
Missionary Position 101, 104
monks 17
Mounting of an Ass 111
movement 23, 28, 29, 46, *89*
mudras 24, 100
Muladhara (First Gate) root
    chakra 17, 20, 23, *34*, 36,
    37, 39, 62
multiple orgasms 8–9, 19,
    20, 23, 59, 71, 77, 95,
    95, 97, *97*, 106, 114,
    123, *123*
music 20, 46, 50, 84, 89, 97
muslin 82

nadis 17, 24, 33, *33*, 90
nail brush 60
nails 60, 89
neck 57, 62, *62*, 74
Nine Basic Principles 27
    breathing 28, 30–32
    mantras 28, 32–3
    massage 28, 49–50, *50*
    meditation 28, 29–30
    movement 28, 46, *46*
    rituals 28–9
    touch 28, 49, *49*
    visualization 28, 33, *33*,
        34, 36–7
    yoga 28, 41–5
nipples 57, 63, *63*, 69, 74,
    83, 89, 94, 106, 115, 117
nose 62

oils 50, 59, 77, 84, *86*, 90,
    91, 94, 97, 111
om mani padme aum mantra
    23, 32–3
oral sex 14, 109, *109*, 110
orgasm
    controlling 114–15
        pelvic tilt exercises 116
    extended 122, 124
    G-spot 123
    whole-body 122
orgasm stage 69, 70, *70*, 71,
    114, 115, 117, 119, 120
orgasms, multiple *see*
    multiple orgasms
oysters 84

pain and pleasure 92
Pair of Tongs 106, *109*
peace 13, 24
pelvic tilt exercises 116
penetrative sex 10, *11*, 49,
    68, 70, 74, 77, 94

penis 57, 59, 68, 69, 72, 74, 104, 106, 110, 117, 123
squeeze technique 77
see also lingam
performance fears 74
perfume/scent 20, 32, 82, 89, *89*
perineum 20, 37, 39, 121, *122*
pillows 82, 89, 103, 110, 111
plateau stage 69, 70, 114, 115, 117, 119, 120
pleasure of the moment 8–9, *9*
point of ejaculatory inevitability 119
pomegranates 84
potpourri 82
prakriti (female principle) 100
prana 16, 39, *39*
premature ejaculation 55
preparing yourself 86, *86*, 89
Pressed Position 103, *103*
Pressing Position 100, 103, *103*
pressure 74, *74*
prolonging the sex act 14, 15, 19, 77, *77*
squeeze technique 77
puberty 55
pubic hair 90
pulse 69
purusha (male principle) 100

rear-entry positions 110–11, *110*
refractory period 115, 123
relationships 9–10, 27, 28, 54, 81, 124
relaxation 97
techniques 29
resolution stage 69, 114, 115, 120
riding the tiger 24, *24*
riding the wave 95, 97, 124, *124*
rituals 28–9
rose petals 85
Rubbing of a Boar 111

sacred spot 123
Sahasrara (Seventh Gate) crown chakra 17, 20, 36, 37, 39, 105
samadhi (sense of bliss) 16, 17
scrotum 57, 64, 117
self discipline 23
self-exploration 55–7, *56*, 117, *117*
focused 57–9
self-expression 81
self-knowledge 54, 55
self-pleasuring 58–9, *68*
see also masturbation
semen 19, 20, 119
sensate focus 74, 77
caressing 74
soul-gazing 74
senses 20, *20*, 60, 81
sensuality 82

setting the scene 80–85
accessories and oils 84–5
candlelight 82–4, *83*
flowers and fragrance 82
the foods of love 84, *85*
sensuality and spirituality 82
sex as a celebration 7–8
sex play 49
sex positions 94, *95*, 99–111
face to face: man on top 101
churning 104
Clasping Position 100, *100*, 101
Fixing a Nail 103
Mare's Position 103
Missionary Position 104
variations 103
Pressed Position 103
Pressing Position 100, 103, *103*
Splitting of a Bamboo 100, 103, *103*
Widely Open Position 103
'Y' position 101, *104*
Yawning Position 103
face to face: side by side 105
Twining Position 105, *105*
face to face: upright positions 105–6
Supported Congress 106, *106*
Suspended Congress 106, *106*
face to face: woman on top 106
Pair of Tongs 106, *109*
oral sex 109–10
Mouth Congress 109, *109*
soixante-neuf ('69') 110
rear-entry 110–11, *110*
Congress of an Elephant 100, 111, *111*
Congress of a Cat 111
Jump of a Tiger 111
Mounting of an Ass 111
Rubbing of a Boar 111
sexual ecstasy 14, 49, *49*, 80
controlled 95, 114–15
pelvic tilt exercises 116
hours of pleasure 124, *124*
knowing when to stop 119
knowing your trigger points 117, *117*, 119
stopping ejaculation 120
delaying tactics 120–21
types of orgasm
G-spot orgasms 123
multiple orgasms 123
whole-body and extended orgasms 122

sexual response cycle 114
arousal or excitement stage 69, 70, 71, 74, 114, 115, 120
being in tune 70–71
orgasm stage 69, 70, *70*, 71, 114, 115, 117, 120
plateau stage 69, 70, 114, 115, 117, 119, 120
resolution stage 69, 114, 115, 120
sexual touching 60, 62–4
Shakti 11, 15, 18, 41, 46, 91, 94, 100, 106
sharing 59
Shiva 11, 15, 18, 41, 46, *46*, 91, 94, 100, 106
shoulders 62, *62*
showers 85, 89, 111
silk 59, 77, 91
'69' 110
Sixty-Four Arts 20, *20*, 23, *23*, 46, 80, 81
smell 60
soaps 84, *86*, 89, 111
soixante-neuf 110
soul-gazing 74, 83, *89*, 90, 92
sound 32, 60
spanking 92
spiritual enlightenment 14, *14*, 15
spirituality 82
Splitting of a Bamboo 100, 103, *103*
sponges 59, 60, 84, 91
squeeze technique 77
Sting 6
Supported Congress 106, *106*
Suspended Congress 106, *106*
Svadhisthana (Second Gate) chakra 17, 20, 23, 37, 39, 63

taking your time 92
Tantra: meaning of the word 10
Tantric Sex Ritual 20, 28–9, 79–97, 114
beginning the ritual 89–91
massage and visualization 90–91
being within 94
Coming from Behind 110
variations 110–11
eternal changes 111
games to play 94
the language of touch 91–2
pain and pleasure 92
taking your time 92
Mouth Congress 109–10, *109*
preparing yourself 86, *86*, 89
relax and chill out 97, *97*
riding the wave 97, 99
setting the scene 81–5
accessories and oils 84–5

candlelight 82–4, *83*
flowers and fragrance 82
the foods of love 84, *85*
sensuality and spirituality 82
tantrikas (practitioners of Tantra) 7, 8, 13, 14, 15, 17, 19, 23, 24, 28, 41, 49, 82, 92, 99, 123
taste 60, *60*
tattoos, temporary 89–90
teenagers 55
teeth 77, 92, *92*
tension 62, *62*
testicles 69
Theosophica Practica 16
thighs 58
toes 57, 64, 74, 105
tongue 77, 91, 97
touch 28, 29, *39*, 49, *49*, 60, 74, *74*, 89, 91, *92*, 97
pain and pleasure 92
taking your time 92
towels 59, 84, 119
Tree Pose 45
trigger points 117, *117*
triggers of arousal and stimulation 66, 68
Turned Shiva Posture 45
Twining Position 105, *105*

undressing 91, *91*

vagina 37, 39, 69, 84, 103, 104, 106, 110, 117, 119, 123
see also yoni
vaporizers 32
Vatsyayana 15–16, 20, 23, 46, 80, 81, 82, 84, 92, 97, 100, 103–6, 109, 111
velvet 77
Vishnu 15
Vishuddi (Fifth Gate) chakra 17, 37, 39, 62
visualization 23, 28, 33, *33*, 34, 39, 90, 95, 122

washing 86
whole body awareness *29*
whole-body orgasm 122
Widely Open Position 103

'Y' position 101, *104*
yang energy 20
yantras 41
Yawning Position 103, *103*
yin energy 20
yoga 17, 28
Corpse Pose 45
The Cat Stretch 44
The Cobra 42, *42*
The Lotus 41
Tree Pose 43
Turned Shiva Posture 43
yoni 8, 23, 32, 33, 64, 72, 94, 104, 106
see also vagina

AROMATHERAPY AND CANDLE SUPPLIERS

UK

G Baldwin & Co
171–173 Walworth Road
Elephant and Castle
London SE17 1RW
020 7703 5550

Neal's Yard Remedies
26–34 Ingate Place
Battersea
London SW8 3NS
for Mail Order Catalogue
ring 01618 317875
mail@nealsyardremedies.com

Tisserand Aromatherapy
Newtown Road
Hove
Sussex BN3 7BA
for Mail Order Catalogue
ring 01273 325666
info@avalonnaturalproducts.com

Fleur Aromatherapy
Langston Priory Mews
Kingham
Oxon OX7 6UP
01608 659909
sales@fleur.co.uk

Norfolk Essential Oils
Pates Farm
Tipsend
Welney
Wisbech PE14 9SQ
01354 638065
sales@neoils.demon.co.uk

Audrey Leigh Essential Oils
60 Mold Road
Connahs Quay
Deeside
Flintshire CH5 4QN
mike@audreyleigh.com

The Body Jewellery Shop
239 Station Road
Harrow
Middlesex HA1 2TB
020 8424 9000
info@bodyjewelleryshop.co.uk

Shop 4 Essential Oils Ltd
P O Box 45
Uttoxeter
Staffordshire
West Midlands ST14 8BR
0800 0180528
info@shop4essentialoils.com

USA

Neal's Yard Remedies
79 East Putnam Avenue
Greenwich, CT 06830–5644
888 697 8721 (888 NYR USA1)
nealsyardremedies@yahoo.com

Amet's Essentials
9311 Piscataway Road
Clinton, MD 20735
877 328 6663
essentials@amets.net

Celestial Touch
P.O. Box 9338
Marina Del Rey, CA 90295
877 81 AROMA
celestialtch@earthlink.net

Aroma-Pure
P.O. Box 1337
American Fork, UT 84003
888 826 2486
aroma-pure@juno.com

Aromatherapy Outlet
P.O. Box 4057
Hialeah, FL 33014
305 828 7655
info@aromatherapyoutlet.com

AromaWerks
P.O. Box 67066
Albuquerque, NM 87193
505 890 1110
info@aromawerks.com

Birch Hill Happenings
2898 County Road 103
Barnum, MN 55707–8808
218 384 9294
albuddy1@aol.com

Enfleurage
321 Bleecker Street
New York, NY 10014
888 387 0300
oils@enfleurage.com

Florapathics
P.O. Box 66723
Houston, TX 77266
832 467 4900
service@florapathics.com

Mountain Rose Herbs
85472 Dilley Lane
Eugene, OR 97405
800 879 3337
info@mountainroseherbs.com

One Planet
10247 E. Convington Street
Tucson, AZ 85748
877 259 6392
oneplanet@oneplanetnatural.com

Samara Botane
300 Queen Anne Avenue N. #378
Seattle, WA 98109
800 782 4532
samara@wingedseed.com

Stress Dynamics
2877 Happy Valley Circle
Newnan, GA 30263–4065
770 502 3716
mercedes@stressdynamics.com

Terra Soleil Ltd.
P.O. Box 12
Gardiner, NY 12525
845 256 1294
karen@terrasoleil.com

Touched By A Scent
2633 South Hampton Road
Ownsboro, KY 42303–9541
866 428 4469
info@TBAScent.com

Truess
P.O. Box 540542
North Salt Lake, UT 84054–0542
801 936 0308
n.orders@truess.com

Whiffs True Aromatherapy
70 Lakeshore Lane
Chattanooga, TN 37415
877 519 7745
whiffs@whiffs.com

The publishers would like to thank the following sources for their kind permission to reproduce the pictures in this book:

AKG London: 7, /Jean-Louis Nou: 18

Axiom Photographic Agency Ltd/ Chris Caldicott: 14

The Bridgeman Art Library: 16 left

Imagebank: 36

Werner Forman Archive: 3, 4–5, 6